THE PEDIATRIC NURSE PRACTITIONER

THE PEDIATRIC NURSE PRACTITIONER

Fernando J. deCastro, M.D., M.P.H., F.A.A.P., F.A.P.H.A.

Assistant Professor of Pediatrics and Community Medicine,
St. Louis University; Director of Ambulatory Pediatric Services,
Cardinal Glennon Memorial Hospital for Children,
St. Louis, Missouri

Ursula T. Rolfe, B.A., M.D.

Assistant Professor of Pediatrics and Community Medicine,
St. Louis University; Associate Director of Ambulatory Pediatric Services,
Cardinal Glennon Memorial Hospital for Children,
St. Louis, Missouri

THE C. V. MOSBY COMPANY

SAINT LOUIS 1972

Printed in the United States of America

International Standard Book Number 0-8016-1220-9

Library of Congress Catalog Card Number 73-176388

Distributed in Great Britain by Henry Kimpton, London

PREFACE

A pediatric nurse practitioner is a registered nurse who has completed an action-oriented training program in ambulatory pediatrics—a pediatric setting geared to care for the nonhospitalized pediatric patient.

The shortage of pediatric health manpower and the need to improve the delivery of health care to children require no discussion. There is a need for doctors and even a greater need for nurses. However, a pediatric nurse practitioner program does not remove nurses from nursing but allows them to enlarge their knowledge and confidence in order to function more effectively in a primary care pediatric ambulatory setting.

There are numerous programs training pediatric nurse practitioners in the United States, some training nurses who are not employed while they are attending the program and some geared only for nurses who are fully employed at the time.

This manual is intended as an outline to allow nurses to expand their empirical knowledge of ambulatory pediatrics by an orderly exposure to its different aspects. It is also intended as a guide which recent pediatric nurse practitioner graduates can consult while gaining experience and confidence in ambulatory pediatrics during the resolution of their re-orientation from a dependent nurse's role to more independent members of a team delivering health care to children.

This manual is further intended as a reference for public health nurses and nurses working in a doctor's office who have never received formal training as pediatric nurse practitioners but have been functioning as such.

We would like to acknowledge first Dr. Arthur E. McElfresh, Chairman of the Department of Pediatrics, St. Louis University. Without Dr. McElfresh's thorough critical review of the manuscript, help, and encouragement this book could not have been accomplished.

We would like to thank Mr. Christo Popoff for the medical illustrations, Miss Patricia Madden and Miss Katherine Bonnot for typing the manuscript, and Sister Marie Weiss for her help in organizing the pediatric nurse practitioner course in our hospital.

Finally, one cannot write a book about pediatric nurse practitioners without acknowledging Dr. Henry K. Silver for his pioneer work in this field; his work has inspired us.

Fernando J. deCastro

Ursula T. Rolfe

CONTENTS

SECTION II **CLINICAL PROBLEMS**

Chapter 1
INTRODUCTION

Pediatrics is the medical specialty concerned with the health of children. As are the other medical specialties, pediatrics is of fairly recent development. In other times and societies the care of children was assumed by general physicians for acute illnesses, and by midwives, grandmothers, and other elderly women members of the extended family for health supervision and counseling.

The gradual disappearance of the extended family, coupled with the development of medical specialties, has been responsible for the development of pediatrics as we know it today.

Pediatrics today is concerned not only with the treatment of acute illnesses in children and with providing comprehensive care during illnesses, but also with health supervision and counseling in order to give every child the conditions for growth and development that will permit each young individual to reach adulthood in his optimum state of physical, mental, and social development. Pediatric practitioners need to understand children as individuals different from adults and as members of their times and of their community. This is both an enormous and an immensely rewarding task. Children are people with infinite and multifaceted needs, and they are also the builders of the future.

Children, as is quite well known, are not just "small adults"; at different ages they have unique anatomic, physiologic, behavioral, and pathologic characteristics.

Anatomically, important variants include thickness of the chest wall, position of the heart, and separation of cranial bones. The chest wall in children is thinner than in adults and, therefore, breath and heart sounds can be heard more easily than in adults. The heart changes from a more horizontal position in infancy to a more vertical position in later childhood; the cranial bones in young children are separated, leaving sutures and fontanels open, rather than being closed as in adults.

Physiologically, children have, relative to their weight, greater caloric needs than adults; the liver and kidney of newborns do not function as well and cannot handle certain medications as well as the adult organs can. Normal variations in growth and height rate, for example, allow children to lose their "baby fat" between the ages of 2 and 5 years.

There are numerous behavioral factors. For example, children go through a period of psychologic negativism between the ages of 18 months and 3 years. As the term implies, children are extremely negative during this stage of development.

Pathologically, children respond to illness differently from adults. For example, children have fewer antibodies because they have not yet had many infectious experiences. They are therefore more susceptible than adults to infectious diseases such as measles or mumps.

Not only must pediatric nurse practitioners realize that children are not small adults, but they must also be aware of community realities. They must accurately weigh the importance of childhood problems and diseases at a particular time in a particular population. For example, in the United States at the beginning of the twentieth century pediatrics was concerned with the high infant mortality, which was largely due to infectious diseases. With wider scientific knowledge, wider distribution of health services, and changes in social conditions, infant mortality has decreased from 200 per 1,000 live births in 1900 to 23 per 1,000 live births today. The control of diarrhea with dehydration and the control of infectious diseases have been responsible to a great extent for the decrease in infant mortality in the United States and other developed countries. Progress in the control of infectious diseases has diminished both infant and childhood mortality. Because of this change pediatrics has become involved with childhood accidents, malignant diseases, and congenital anomalies.

Although scientific progress in the care of children has been great, distribution of medical care is considerably inadequate even in highly developed countries such as the United States. Neonatal mortality, a useful indicator of quality and distribution of medical care, has shown great improvement in the so-called developed countries. In the so-called developing countries malnutrition, diarrhea and dehydration, and other diseases are still rampant, and neonatal mortality is very high. Unfortunately, even within the United States there are great discrepancies in infant mortality in different segments of the population. The mortality rate of those living in urban ghettos is much higher than the rate for wealthier groups.

With the increasing philosophical commitment to total medical care of high quality for every child, physicians and nurses are developing and evaluating more efficient ways to deliver medical care. Since the largest need in medical care is in the area of ambulatory services—less than 10 percent of children receiving medical care need hospitalization—the emphasis has been placed on developing more efficient ways to deliver ambulatory pediatric services. The pediatric nurse practitioner programs can provide such services.

SECTION I
HEALTH APPRAISAL

Chapter 2
THE MEDICAL HISTORY

In numerous pediatric problems the history is the single most important factor in arriving at a correct diagnosis.

Numerous authors have repeatedly stated that history taking is a gift with which certain persons are endowed. Although natural talents are useful, sufficient time, empathy, and training to communicate will yield accurate and satisfactory histories. Histories must be clearly and systematically recorded so that the patient's medical chart will be complete for further references.

This chapter will cover the process of obtaining a complete history as well as its correct recording.

HISTORY TAKING

The aim or purpose of the medical history is to learn about symptoms, their nature, and their history; in other words, the history is concerned with the occurrence and chronology of symptoms. Thoroughness and patience will enable the examiner to obtain complete information; training and practice will help him distinguish the relevant from the irrelevant. For example, an 8-year-old child may be brought to the clinic with a history of recurrent abdominal pain that has been occurring since the beginning of the school year. In such a case, extensive dietary details may be irrelevant, but a history of school attendance may be highly relevant and must therefore be patiently and thoroughly pursued.

In the process of history taking the examiner needs (1) to observe the patient and his parents, and (2) to be an active listener.

Before observations and actual history taking begin, it is necessary that there be a good physical and psychologic setting. There should be as much privacy as possible. A good history is not obtained in a hospital corridor. Psychologically, it is important that a good relationship between the patient and the examiner be established. A few casual remarks regarding a toy the child may have brought or a particular sport in which the child is interested can do wonders in relaxing the atmosphere of the examining room.

In observing the patient and his family the examiner may find many nonverbal clues of significance. The physical appearance of the family may tell more about their nutritional status than a dietary history. The attitudes of the family members toward each other—looks, gestures—may reveal much

5

about the emotional status of the family. In the case of an infant who does not use words, it is especially important to look for nonverbal signs of contentment or of unhappy home situations.

Above all, the examiner, in order to obtain an accurate history, needs to be an interested active listener.

The examiner should be aware of certain techniques that will help elicit extensive and meaningful information. He should give special consideration to (1) vocabulary, (2) type of questions, (3) verbal aids to communication, and (4) nonverbal aids to communication.

The vocabulary used in taking the history is extremely important. The examiner must quickly establish the level of verbal understanding of the family so that he may word his questions accordingly. Doubtful words should be defined by both the examiner and the patient or his parents. The examiner must know as exactly as possible what the mother means when she says that the child had "measles three times." When talking with children and adolescents the examiner must keep in mind that children at different ages often have a vocabulary of their own. For example, the word "grass" definitely means different things to children of different ages.

The types of questions asked are also important in history taking. These questions may be direct, open-ended, or leading. Direct questions are quick, obtain a great deal of information, and are useful in yielding specific facts (for example, "How old is your child?"). On the other hand, some topics may require open-ended questions to allow more freedom in answering. When the examiner asks, "Does Johnny have sore throats?" the parent is free to answer yes or no, how many, how often, how severe, and so on, and this allows the examiner to pursue a line that may be richer in information. In other cases a leading question (for example, "How many sore throats has Johnny had since the beginning of school?") may be more helpful than either a direct or an open-ended question. However, leading questions are to be handled with care since they may bias the patient into providing false information that he assumes will please the examiner. Several aids make questions more effective. Repetition of the same question with a different inflection on a significant word or phrase may prove quite revealing. Answering a patient's question with another question such as, "Why do you ask?" will often elicit spontaneous, helpful answers from the patient.

In addition to the exclusively verbal means of communication, there are also nonverbal means that may facilitate or hinder communication. Making eye contact with the patient will show interest from the examiner and will most likely increase the amount of information obtained from the patient; however, showing distress when a mother says that she spanks her 2-year-old every time he does not eat well may antagonize the mother and hinder further communication.

Some other difficulties that may prevent the flow of communication between the patient and the examiner are to be found in (1) the triangular relationship specific to pediatrics—examiner, parent, and child; (2) anxiety on the part of the examiner; (3) negative attitudes on the part of the patient; and (4) premature offer of advice by the examiner.

In pediatrics, history taking involves a triangular relationship—examiner, parents, and child. Although this triangular participation is essential, it also brings problems of which the examiner needs to take notice. Some of these problems are related to the parents' observation, the parents' possible distortion of facts, and the parents' ability to communicate.

Some parents are unbelievably poor observers of their children. They often miss obvious problems such as moderate and even severe deafness in their children. In certain situations, because of parental problems, the facts are consciously or subconsciously distorted. For example, the parents of a mentally retarded child often lead the interviewer to believe that the child is of normal intelligence. Finally, other parents simply lack the ability to verbally express what they have observed in their children.

Certain people or certain topics, because of the examiner's own background, may arouse anxiety in the examiner and communication will tend to diminish. For example, an overprotective mother may disturb an examiner and make him anxious. If his anxiety becomes evident, communication with that mother will diminish. It is the patient's or his parents' privilege to be anxious. Expression of anxiety by the examiner will produce conflict with the patient and may render the examiner considerably less effective. Also some feelings in the patient may, in a way, prove contagious to the examiner and become roadblocks in history taking. Of these transferred feelings, anger is the most common. An angry patient may in turn arouse the examiner to anger, and history taking will be impaired. The examiner must remain in control of himself and the situation at all times and must not allow his own background or the patient's negative feelings to deviate him from his goal.

Finally, the examiner should be aware of the fact that he should not give advice while he is obtaining the history. Premature offer of advice to the patient again creates the possibility of diminished communication.

The medical history provides not only a tremendous source of information, but also is often a therapeutic means in itself. By simply coherently explaining his complaints, the patient and the family may realize their problem. A diet recall may by itself make a mother see that her child is eating more candy than she realized. Relating chronologically the occurrence of abdominal pain with school absenteeism may be the beginning of the realization of the mechanism of a school phobia.

A good physical and psychologic atmosphere for the patient, together with an interested, positive, clever examiner will produce a complete and thorough history. Since a complete history is essential in the diagnosis and treatment of the patient, its importance should be greatly emphasized.

HISTORY RECORDING

Orderly and systematic recording of a medical history is essential. The patient's record is the source to which several members of the health team will refer on numerous occasions. To each one of them the history should provide as much information as possible, and this information must be made accessible by clarity and order of recording.

Many institutions use an outline or "check-out" history while others provide no specific structure. However, the format at all institutions is usually similar, thus facilitating communication among health professionals regarding a patient.

The subsequent outline should be adapted to the age of the child and the condition for which he is brought to the health care facility. A complete history of a child often consists of the following sections:

Identifying data	Past medical history
Chief complaint (CC)	Family history
Present illness (PI)	Personality history
Prenatal and neonatal history	Social history
Developmental history	Habits
Nutritional history	Review of systems
Immunization history	

Identifying data. The initial part of the history includes name, address, telephone number, sex, date and place of birth, source of referral, parental occupation, insurance, and hospital or clinic number, if applicable. Most clinics incorporate this information into clinic cards and stamps. A statement of the examiner's opinion of the reliability of the informant, as well as the informant's relationship to the patient, should be included.

Chief complaint (CC). The chief complaint consists of the patient's or his parents' brief account of the problem that brings him to seek medical help and its duration. It should be recorded in one sentence (for example, "Earache since yesterday.").

Present illness (PI). The present illness is a chronologic account of what has happened to the patient since he was well. One to three paragraphs should accurately cover the development of the present illness.

The duration of the illness, is, of course, important and the description of the present illness usually starts with a statement of duration. For example, "This child was well until 3 months of age" or "until 3 days prior to admission." The interviewer must avoid the use of days of the week or months when stating the duration of illness, since the history may be read years later.

Pertinent negative findings should also be recorded. For example, for a child who has rheumatic heart disease in which tolerance to exercises may be impaired, it is important to state that the patient has "no intolerance to exercise." As the interviewers gain in medical knowledge, they will be better prepared to record pertinent negative findings.

Table 1. Apgar score*

Sign	0	1	2
Heart rate	Absent	Below 100	Over 100
Respiratory efforts	Absent	Slow, irregular	Good, crying
Muscle tone	Limp	Some flexion	Active motion
Response to catheter in nostril	No response	Grimace	Cough or sneeze
Color	Blue, pale	Body pink, extremities blue	Completely pink

*From Apgar, V.: Cur. Res. Anesth. Analges. 32:260, 1953.

Prenatal and neonatal history. Prenatal and neonatal history is particularly important in infants and toddlers and includes length of gestation as well as maternal health and history of drug ingestion during pregnancy. The history must include duration of labor, complications, type of anesthesia used at delivery, maternal complications, birth weight, and need for resuscitation. The status of the infant at birth and 5 minutes later is often summarized by an Apgar Score (Table 1). Neonatal history reveals abnormalities during the first month of life including need of incubator, jaundice, and feeding patterns. In obtaining the neonatal history it is useful to find out whether or not the child went home with the mother after birth. Although most important in infants and toddlers, the prenatal and neonatal history is also of importance in older children and adolescents with specific problems. For example, in dealing with an older child or adolescent who has cerebral palsy or epileptic seizures this part of the history is very significant.

Developmental history. The history of developmental milestones is an important way to evaluate brain development. It should be age related. For example, it is pertinent to know when a 2-year-old first sat unsupported, talked, and walked, or when a four-year-old first talked, his vocabulary at 18 months, and when he first used sentences. However, these items become irrelevant in an 8-year-old who is doing well in the third grade. Items commonly assessed with their average age of performance are shown in Table 2 and are discussed in Chapter 6. These are relatively age specific, easily remembered items for the mother of an infant or toddler. The mother of a 6-year-old may not remember items relating to earlier ages, but will know whether her child is riding a bicycle or not and when he began to ride it. Of course, in older children performance in school becomes more important than a history of the developmental milestones.

Nutritional history. The nutritional history should include whether the baby was breast fed or bottle fed. If he was bottle fed, the record must include details of the formula. Nutritional history also includes vitamin intake, fluoridation of the water, age of introduction of solid foods, and eating habits. The nutritional history should also be age related. For example, a detailed nutritional history of early infancy is unimportant in a ten-year-old who is growing well, but it is very important in a one-year-old who is failing to thrive.

Immunizations. The section on immunizations consists of the history of inoculations received, including type, number, reaction, and date. This section of the history also includes the history of tuberculin skin testing and other skin testing such as histoplasmin (see Chapter 8).

Past history. In the section of past history, the examiner asks questions regarding (1) allergies, (2) medications, (3) past illnesses, (4) operations, (5) hospitalization, and (6) accidents. The allergic history includes questions related to asthma, hay fever, eczema and, most importantly, the history of any previous drug reaction. In the medication history, past significant medications are recorded (for example, whether the patient has been on steroids or not). In the past history of illnesses, the examiner records the history of infectious diseases, convulsions, or any illness for which the child has required hospitalization. Any other severe disease should also be recorded. The dates and outcome of these illnesses are important. Finally, this part of the history must include the date, type, extent, and permanent effect of any accidents or operations.

Family history. In the section on family history the examiner finds out parental age, health, and marital status, the health of siblings and immediate relatives, and the cause of death in any of the above-mentioned relatives. This section also covers the history in the family of heart disease, diabetes, tuberculosis, congenital anomalies, high blood pressure, kidney disease, epilepsy or seizure disorder, mental retardation, deafness, and other illnesses. Positive findings need to be pursued further. For example, if the family history shows that the father died at age 35 of a heart attack, the interviewer must make further efforts to determine if heart attack caused the death of any more distant relatives.

Personality history. In the personality history the examiner evaluates the patient's relationship with parents, siblings, and schoolmates. It should, as always in pediatrics, be age related and problem specific. For example, school progress is very important in school-age children because it tells the examiners about the child's social functioning. The history of bowel and bladder training is very important in preschool children because it tells the examiner about the mother-child relationship. Bladder and bowel training history is much less important in a 10-year-old who is doing well in school and is well adapted otherwise. It may, however, be very relevant in a 10-year-old child with constipation (see Chapters 6 and 15).

Social history. The social history appraises the family's social environment. Family income, home size, number of rooms, sleeping facilities, heating, sewerage, and water facilities are all important. For example, lead poisoning is associated with living in old homes built before World War II that are in poor state of repair. In these homes, children often eat paint chips containing lead that fall off the walls. In the social history the family social adaptation is important. For example, a family where the father works every day and does not drink and a family where the father is an alcoholic without a permanent job offer striking contrasts in their social adaptation.

Habits. The section on habits includes eating, sleeping, and toilet habits, as well as other habits such as enuresis, encopresis, masturbation, thumb sucking, nail biting, breath-holding spells, and temper tantrums. As previously stated a bowel and bladder training history may give the examiner an insight into the mother-child relationship. It may also reveal the background of a particular symptom such as stubbornness, which, according to psychoanalytic theory, is associated with developmental emotional arrest at the anal stage where most children are normally stubborn.

Review of systems (ROS). In the review of systems significant symptoms related to illnesses in each organ system are asked in an orderly way as follows:

Head, eyes, ears, nose, and throat—frequent colds, stuffy nose, postnasal drip, mouth breathing, ear infection, epistaxis

Cardiorespiratory—dyspnea, cyanosis, wheezing, chronic cough, previous pneumonia

Gastrointestinal—appetite, feeding problems, vomiting, diarrhea, constipation, encopresis, abdominal pain, jaundice

Genitourinary—enuresis, frequency and dysuria, urinary tract infection, vaginal discharge, menses

Neuromuscular—headaches, nervousness, dizziness, seizures, joint pain, unsteadiness, frequent falls, loss of consciousness

Special senses—hearing, vision, need for glasses

General—weight gain or loss, fatigue, skin color

The interviewer should record the history in the above order, although, depending on the situation, certain parts could be omitted and certain other parts expanded. For example, a child first seen for a seizure disorder needs a complete history and physical examination with a detailed neurologic examination. On the other hand, a one-paragraph interval history may be all that is necessary for a child who is followed regularly at the health facility.

Chapter 3

THE PHYSICAL EXAMINATION

The physical examination is an important diagnostic tool in the health evaluation of both asymptomatic or seemingly well children and symptomatic or sick children. It also provides an excellent opportunity for patient-examiner interaction, which should be utilized to its maximum potential.

There are four basic techniques used during the performance of a physical examination:

1. Inspection
2. Palpation
3. Percussion
4. Auscultation

In other words, first look at the patient (inspection), then touch him (palpation), then tap him (percussion), and lastly, listen to him (auscultation).

This chapter will be divided into two parts: perspectives of the physical examination and its recording and specific techniques utilized in examining different parts of the body.

PERSPECTIVES

A gentle, considerate approach to the patient is of utmost importance. The small infant or child may first be examined in his mother's lap. Allowing the young patient to view the instrument that will be used—for example, dangling the stethoscope in front of a baby or demonstrating the otoscope for the toddler ("see my little light, I am going to shine it into your ear")—will often do much to allay the child's fear. At times, the mother may be instructed to demonstrate certain signs. The apprehensive toddler may refuse to flex his neck for the examiner but will do so readily for his mother. When examining older children, the examiner must explain all procedures in simple terms and should warn the child if the procedure will be painful or uncomfortable. Only in this way will the child be able to develop trust in the examiner.

Forceful restraint should be used only when absolutely essential, and then only the minimal amount of restraint consistent with safety and adequacy of examination. For example, a small child's ears can usually be examined best by having the child sit in his mother's lap with his head immobilized against the mother's chest. This type of restraint is obviously much less frightening than the time-honored procedure of immobilizing the child on the examining table with his head pinned between his forcefully extended arms.

In pediatrics the examiner must be opportunistic during the examination—doing that which is least upsetting and for which he needs the cooperation of the patient first, and only at the end doing those parts that will most upset the patient. For example, the examiner should not look at the throat first because it is very upsetting to most children and they will then be crying when the time comes to auscultate the heart.

Although the examination may be performed in the order best suited to the particular child and specific circumstances, recording the findings of the physical examination should be done in an orderly, systematic fashion, essentially from head to toe. Order in recording not only prevents omissions but also, as in the case of the history, facilitates future reviewing of the medical chart.

A complete physical examination of a child should consist of the following sections recorded in the following order:

Vital signs	Ears
Measurements	Neck
General appearance	Thorax
Skin	Lungs
Lymph nodes	Heart
Head	Abdomen
Eyes	Genitalia
Nose	Rectum
Mouth	Extremities
Throat	Neurologic examination

A child does not need a complete physical examination every time he comes to the health care facility. The patient should have a complete physical examination during the first evaluation and at scheduled intervals thereafter. When a child is brought for an acute illness or for follow-up care of an acute or chronic illness, a complete examination is often not done in detail. At such time examination is primarily geared to the organ system involved in the specific illness, although a quick evaluation of the other organ systems may be done as well.

PERFORMANCE

As previously stated the four basic techniques of physical examination are inspection, palpation, percussion, and auscultation. The examiner will use one or a combination of these techniques when examining different regions of the body. Since different sections of the physical examination present specific difficulties, each section will be discussed as a unit.

Vital signs. Vital signs are well known to nurses and include temperature, pulse rate, respiratory rate, and blood pressure.

Children's temperatures are normally higher than those of adults. Usually, rectal temperatures below 100.5° F. are not considered fever in children.

The nurse practitioner obtains the pulse rate in older children, as in adults, by palpation at the wrist. In infants, the pulse rate is often obtained by auscultation of the heart. The normal pulse rate in children is faster than in adults. At birth the normal pulse rate is from 120 to 140. In older children it decreases to the adult rate of 70 to 90. There are numerous causes which may produce variation in pulse rate. Fever and apprehension, as well as heart failure, may cause an increase in pulse rate. A decreased pulse rate is usually found in athletes in training and also in heart block, which may be caused by a congenital heart defect or by digitalis intoxication.

Observation of the child's chest will indicate the respiratory rate. The rate is normally faster in infants than in older children. A fast respiratory rate may simply be due to fever, anxiety, or excitement, but may also indicate heart failure, pneumonia, asthma, or other illnesses reducing oxygenation.

Blood pressure is usually obtained by the auscultatory method in older children; however, in infants the auscultatory method is difficult and blood pressure is most frequently obtained either by palpation or by the flush technique (Chapter 14). The younger the infant, the lower the normal blood pressure. A normal blood pressure in a newborn is about 70 systolic and 40 diastolic. From these low values, the blood pressure increases to adult levels of 120 systolic and 80 diastolic during adolescence.

Measurements. Measurements, for the most part, are unique to pediatrics and are essential in the physical examination of children, since chronically ill children do not grow well. Commonly used body measurements are height, weight, head circumference, and chest circumference (see Chapter 5).

The circumference of the head is measured at its greatest diameter and that of the chest at the level of the nipple line. The head and chest circumferences are of importance during the first year of life when the head is growing at its fastest rate. At birth the head circumference should be at least equal to the chest circumference (see Chapter 5).

It is important to compare the body measurements (height, weight, head circumference, and chest circumference) of a child with those of his peers by utilizing standard charts (see Chapter 5) in order to establish whether or not the child is growing well.

General appearance. The examiner evaluates the child's state of consciousness. *Coma* is an alteration of the state of consciousness indicating prolonged and profound unconsciousness; the patient responds only to deep pain. *Stupor* is a state of unconsciousness in which the child may be momentarily aroused. *Delirium* is a state of confusion, disorientation, irrationality, and, at times, excitability. The examiner must also establish the patient's psychic state (depressed or anxious), his degree of activity (normal or hyperactive), and his state of nutrition (well nourished, thin, or obese). This part of the record must include a general evaluation of the patient's state of development, as compared to his peers both physically and psychologically. For example, in describing a normal 10-year-old one may write, "This is a well-developed, well-nourished 10-year-old who is friendly and cooperative, neatly dressed and appears well."

Skin. The examiner can tell the patient's state of hydration by examination of the skin. The examiner also looks for the presence of eruption or edema and any suggestion of heart disease or anemia. Blood clotting abilities may also be indicated by the skin.

Turgor means fullness and is a term used in relationship to fullness of the skin. A loss of skin turgor is the loss of the normal fullness of the skin that accompanies dehydration. The skin of an infant with normal skin turgor, when pinched, will quickly return to its previous position. In a dehydrated infant, as in a normal adult, skin, when pinched, returns slowly to its original position.

Many diseases such as measles, scarlet fever, or eczema are characterized by rashes (see Chapter 13).

The examination of the skin also reveals the presence or absence of edema. *Edema* is an excessive accumulation of watery fluid in the tissue spaces. The examiner detects edema by the presence of swelling and a transient depression, referred to as *pit,* when applying pressure. Edema is usually found in the most dependent areas (lower back in infants and legs in older children), and it may be an indication of congestive heart failure or malnutrition. Edema in renal diseases usually occurs around the eyes rather than in the most dependent areas of the body. The examination of the skin may suggest the presence of anemia if the skin color is very pale; heart disease if the patient is cyanotic; and abnormal blood coagulation if there are hemorrhages under the skin such as petechiae or excessive bruising. *Petechiae* are minute hemorrhagic spots of pinpoint to pinhead size in the skin which do not blanch on pressure.

Lymph nodes. Lymph nodes are examined by palpation for location, size, mobility, consistency, and sensitivity to pain. The places where the examiner should usually palpate for lymph nodes are the neck, axilla, and inguinal regions.

In the neck, lymph nodes are palpated below the jaw (the submandibular and submental nodes), in the back of the neck below the ear (the posterior cervical nodes), and behind the ear (posterior auricular nodes).

Enlarged lymph nodes are most commonly caused by infection, and the lymph nodes that are enlarged are those draining the region of the infected areas. For example, when there is an infection of the throat, lymph nodes in the neck are enlarged; if the foot is infected, the inguinal nodes are enlarged. A generalized lymphadenopathy may mean the presence of a malignant disease.

Head. Examination of the head is relevant primarily in infancy, since most of the growth of the head occurs during the first year of life.

The examiner should inspect the head for size (see Chapter 5) and shape.

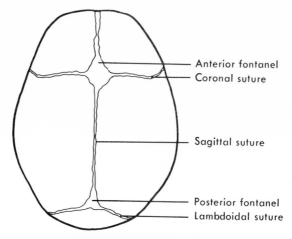

Fig. 1. Top of infant head.

Transient asymmetry or abnormal shape is not uncommon in newborns and is caused by intrauterine positions.

The examination of infants during the first year of life should include palpation of the sutures and fontanels. *Sutures* are the lines between the skull bones. *Fontanels* are one of several membranous intervals at the angle of the cranial bones in infants. Clinically, there are two important ones, anterior and posterior. The anterior fontanel is at the junction of the frontal and parietal bones (Fig. 1). The posterior one is at the junction of the parietal and occipital bones. The posterior fontanel usually closes between birth and 3 months of age and the anterior one between 10 and 16 months of age. The most important fontanel is the anterior, which measures from 0.5 to 2.5 cm in width at birth. Fontanels indicate the degree of intracranial pressure. During dehydration, the fontanels are depressed since the intracranial tension is low. When there is intracranial hypertension, as with hydrocephalus, the fontanels bulge. The fontanels may also bulge when the child is crying, but in this case they retract when crying stops.

Eyes. Examination of the eye consists essentially of four parts: observation of the eye for redness of the conjunctiva or increased lacrimation or tearing; inspection with the help of a penlight to check the pupils and for muscle imbalance; examination with an ophthalmoscope for opacities of the transparent media and the fundus; and determination of visual acuity by simple screening techniques (see Chapter 4).

Redness of the conjunctiva is often caused by conjunctivitis, or pink-eye. Excessive unilateral lacrimation or tearing suggests to the examiner plugging of the nasolacrimal duct, a common condition in young infants.

Inspection of the eye must include examination for pupillary size and

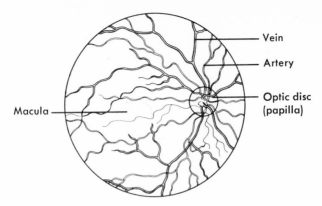

Fig. 2. Fundus of the eye.

reaction to light as well as for strabismus or "squinting." The examiner shines a light 13 to 15 inches away from the child's eye and observes whether or not the light falls in the center of each pupil. Alternately covering each eye while shining the light and watching for motion of the eye is also useful in determining squinting and is called a cover test. This part of the examination must also attempt to detect opacities in the eyes and abnormal jerky movements (nystagmus). Proper function of the eye muscle is determined by having the child follow an object in all directions without moving his head.

Failure to detect abnormalities of muscle balance in the eye early in life (between 3 and 4 years of age) may result in unilateral loss of vision (amblyopia ex anopsia). Since at that early age cooperation from the patient is unfortunately minimal, the examiner must give special attention to this part of the examination. An ophthalmologist should further evaluate the patient if there is paralysis of an eye at any age or inability to fuse or use the two eyes together after the child is 18 months of age.

Examination of the eye with an ophthalmoscope is the most difficult part of the eye examination. It should cover two areas: examination of the transparent media of the eye and examination of the eye ground or fundus. First, select a +8 lens and start the examination approximately 6 inches away from the eye; as one approaches the eye and slowly changes the ophthalmoscope lens toward zero lens, a red reflex becomes apparent through the pupillary opening. Absence of this red reflex indicates opacity of the transparent media of the eye such as in cataracts. Secondly, the fundus itself is seen when the examiner almost touches the eye with the ophthalmoscope while using a 0 to −2 lens. In the fundus (Fig. 2) he looks for abnormalities of the optic disc, such as papilledema, which is indicated by blurring of the disc edges, and for specks of red blood, which indicate retinal hemorrhage. Vision screening will be discussed in Chapter 4.

Nose. The nose is usually inspected for deviation of the septum (the wall separating the two sides of the nose) and for type of drainage. The drainage can be watery, bloody, or thick and yellow (purulent). A chronic, recurrent, watery discharge which comes every year at the same time suggests allergic rhinitis. A unilateral purulent discharge suggests a foreign body on that side of the nose. Epistaxis, or bloody nose, will be discussed in Chapter 12. The examiner must look for patency of the airway by closing the child's mouth and one nostril at a time. Inability of the newborn infant to breathe through his nose may indicate choanal atresia (blockage of the nasal airway).

Mouth. In the examination of the mouth the examiner often overlooks inspection of the teeth for dental caries or cavities and examination of the palate for abnormalities. About half of all 2-year-old children have at least one cavity. The examiner must check for the presence of cleft palate without cleft lip, a finding often missed in examining young infants.

Other findings in the mouth are Epstein pearls in the newborn, Koplik's spots in measles, and swollen gums with vesicles on the tongue and buccal mucosa in herpetic stomatitis. Epstein pearls are white keratin plugs that appear in the palate of newborns; they are insignificant. Koplik's spots are white specks on a reddish blue base most commonly located opposite to the first upper molar. They accompany only measles and are helpful in establishing a diagnosis.

Throat. The examiner must inspect the throat for the condition of the tonsils and epiglottis and must also note and record abnormalities of the voice.

The tonsils need to be examined for size, redness, and the presence of exudate. Red tonsils without exudate suggest a viral pharyngitis. Marked redness with the presence of an exudate would favor a bacterial tonsillitis such as streptococcal pharyngitis. Experience will gradually acquaint the examiner with the normal size of the tonsils at each age.

The epiglottis is normally not visible but in some cases of croup it may be very swollen and it may then appear as a cherry red midline mass. All evaluations of the throat that disclose a cherry red epiglottis suggest the presence of severe bacterial croup, which may produce complete obstruction; in such cases tracheotomy may be necessary.

This part of the physical examination should also cover the presence or absence of hoarseness.

Ears. The ears should be inspected for abnormal position and possible presence of fistula. Low set ears (top of ear below the level of the eye) suggest kidney disease. Fistulas or openings around the ears may be present; these fistulas need to be repaired in order to prevent future infection. The nurse must perform an otoscopic examination of the external canal or passage between the outside and the eardrum, as well as of the tympanic membrane or eardrum. Abnormal redness or exudate in the canal suggests otitis externa.

The canal is often full of cerumen, or wax. In such a case, the wax can either be removed with a curet, or it can be irrigated and flushed out with tepid water. When the tympanic membrane is not perforated it is easier and less traumatic to remove the wax by irrigation. For irrigation, two to three drops of hydrogen peroxide are placed in the canal and after 10 minutes the ear canal is irrigated with tepid water with the help of a syringe. It is important that the water is tepid, since water that is too cold or too warm may produce dizziness. It is less traumatic if a rubber catheter of approximately 1 inch in length is attached to the tip of the syringe.

Figs. 3 and 4 show the appearance of the eardrum (tympanic membrane) and the proper way for a mother to hold her child for an ear examination. The tympanic membrane is usually grayish blue and translucent and with a light reflex going from the umbo anteroinferiorly. The umbo is the point of insertion of the long process of one of the small middle ear bones called the malleus. To observe the tympanic membrane with the otoscope, the examiner should pull the auricle (outside of the ear) upward, outward, and backward in children, and slightly downward in infants. The different methods of examination are necessary because of the different position of the ear canal in children and in infants.

In acute otitis media and in chronic serous otitis media the light reflex becomes distorted because the tympanic membrane is pushed out by fluid. Also the normal translucency and color change, and the tympanic membrane becomes thick and red. Hearing screening tests are discussed in Chapter 4.

Neck. Examination of the neck should reveal abnormal positions, cysts, enlargement of the thyroid or parotid glands, and lymph node abnormalities.

Abnormal positions accompany conditions such as torticollis (wryneck). Further observation and palpation may show cysts along the side of the neck, which are often branchial, or remnants of gills, and which need to be treated by surgery.

The thyroid gland is in the middle of the neck anteriorly, and it should be palpated for enlargement. An enlarged thyroid gland indicates a condition called goiter. The parotid gland sits at the angle of the jaw and should also be palpated. It is enlarged most frequently in mumps. Cervical lymph nodes are palpated for possible enlargement, as previously described.

Thorax. Careful observation and palpation of the thorax may reveal abnormalities. Two common abnormalities of the thorax are beadings along the junctions of the costochondral margins caused by rickets and bulging on the left side caused by an enlarged heart. The breast is observed and palpated in this part of the examination. (See Chapter 17 for discussion of some breast abnormalities.)

Lungs. Before the actual examination of the lungs takes place, the examiner must observe the type of breathing. Breathing may be easy or difficult. Difficult breathing is called dyspnea and is a general term for inspiratory obstruction, expiratory obstruction, and other types of respiratory difficulty. An inspiratory obstruction usually produces an audible high pitched noise—stridor—which

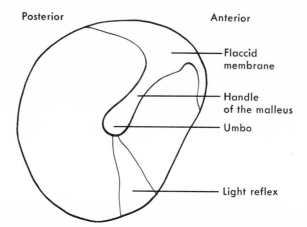

Fig. 3. Tympanic membrane (eardrum).

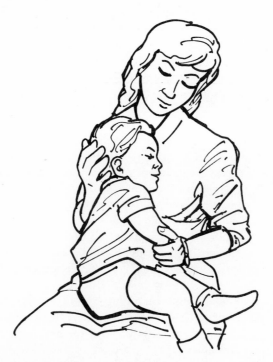

Fig. 4. Mother holding child for ear examination.

is most commonly heard in croup. In expiratory obstructions such as asthma there is a prolonged expiratory phase and wheezing upon auscultation. Dyspnea without either inspiratory or expiratory obstruction can be found in conditions such as congestive heart failure. Intercostal retraction is often associated with dyspnea. Supraclavicular retraction and nasal flaring are often indications of severe dyspnea.

Percussion or tapping helps the examiner to determine disease. Normally the percussion note in a lung full of air is resonant. When there is fluid in the chest, as in pleural effusion, the percussion note becomes flat. In conditions in which there is an increased amount of fluid but the chest is not full of fluid, as in pneumonia, the note is dull. If there is too much air, as in pneumothorax (where there is air between the lung and the chest wall) or in asthma (where there is air trapping in the lung), the note is hyperresonant.

Auscultation allows the examiner to listen to breath sounds. Normal breath sounds are *vesicular,* in which a soft, low pitched sound in inspiration is followed by shorter sounds during expiration; *bronchial* or *tubular,* which are similar to the sounds heard upon auscultating over the larynx during respiration; and *bronchovesicular,* which are a mixture of bronchial and vesicular sounds. Vesicular breath sounds are heard over most of the chest except over the larynx and trachea and in infants over the upper chest. In the upper chest in infants, because of increased transmission, the breath sounds are bronchiovesicular.

In pathologic states one may hear tubular or bronchial breathing over the posterior chest, which means that there is increased transmission between the trachea and the periphery of the chest. This condition occurs when there is solidification or consolidation of a piece of lung, as in pneumonia.

Abnormal sounds heard on auscultation are *ronchi, rales, wheezes,* and *rubs. Ronchi* are loud, gurgling sounds caused by transmitted upper respiratory noises produced by secretions in either the pharynx or trachea. *Rales* are sounds caused by the passage of air through bronchi and alveoli that contain mucus or exudate. Rales are heard in pneumonia. *Wheezes* are high pitched sounds heard on expiration upon auscultation if there is narrowing of the bronchi (for example, in asthma or bronchiolitis). *Rubs* are rubbing sounds similar to the noise made by rubbing two pieces of leather together. Rubs accompany pleural irritation.

Heart. Examination of the heart first reveals movements of the left side of the chest caused by the action of the heart (precordial activity). Precordial activity is related to heart size. For example, a very active chest in front of the heart suggests cardiac enlargement.

The point at which the tip of the heart hits the chest wall, the point of maximal impulse, is important for determining heart size and should also be observed and palpated. It may be outside the nipple line in normal infants, but after infancy it is inside the nipple line at the fifth intercostal space. Failure to feel the point of maximal impulse usually means increased fluid or air between the heart and the chest wall. This may occur in pericarditis or pneumomediastinum. Marked displacement of the point of maximal impulse often means that the heart has been pushed to one side as in pneumothorax. Abnormal turbulence in flow in the heart can be so great that it can be palpated as a *thrill*. Thrills are always an indication of cardiac abnormality.

Upon auscultation of the heart the examiner first evaluates rhythm. Normal rhythm is what is referred to as normal sinus rhythm. In children, the examiner often notices a slight speeding of the heart during inspiration and a slowing of the heart rate during expiration. This is called normal sinus arrhythmia. In pathologic states the rhythm may be too fast (tachycardia) or too slow (bradycardia).

After evaluating the rhythm the examiner must listen to the entire precordium, but especially to the valve areas to evaluate heart sounds and determine the presence of murmurs. *Heart sounds* are normal sounds due to closure of heart valves. The first heart sound is due to closure of the mitral and tricuspid or atrioventricular valves when the heart contracts (systole); the second is due to closure of the pulmonary and aortic valves when the heart relaxes (diastole). In some states, not always pathologic, turbulence in flow in the heart can be heard by auscultation as a *murmur* (Fig. 5). Murmurs should be characterized according to location (where it is best heard), position in the cycle (after the first or the second heart sound), loudness, pitch, and effect of exercise. It is the job of the pediatric nurse practitioner to determine whether a murmur is functional and innocent, or organic (see Chapter 14).

Abdomen. The examination of the abdomen should begin by noticing its size and contour. The presence of either obesity or malnutrition can be determined by observation of the abdomen. In infants the presence of abnormal peristaltic wave or waves, caused by bowel motility, suggests gastrointestinal obstruction such as pyloric stenosis. Further inspection of the abdomen may show the presence of umbilical hernia, which appears as a protruding mass at the navel. Inguinal and femoral hernias may be found in the groin. The former appears as a mass in the groin going into the scrotum. The latter appears as a mass in the mid–upper thigh, immediately below the groin.

The abdomen (Fig. 5) should be palpated for liver, spleen, and abnormal masses. The liver is palpated in the right upper quadrant, below the right rib edge. The liver, when normal in size, is usually not palpated in older children and adolescents. In infants the liver is normally larger, and the edge can usually be palpated 2 to 3 cm below the right costal margin. An enlarged liver accompanies many illnesses, including congestive heart failure.

The spleen is normally not palpated in older children and adolescents. In infants and young children its tip can often be palpated in the left upper quadrant, below the left rib margin. Enlargement of the spleen often accompanies infectious mononucleosis (see Chapter 13) and sickle cell anemia in

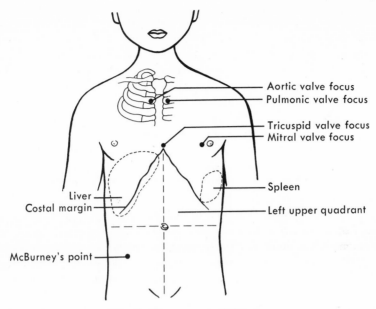

Fig. 5. Thorax and abdomen.

young children. In older children with sickle cell anemia the spleen is not enlarged. The spleen can also be enlarged in malignant diseases, such as leukemia, and in severe infections.

Abnormal masses in the abdomen in children are most commonly retroperitoneal. In other words, they are located against the posterior wall of the abdomen and therefore they are felt by deep palpation of the abdomen. Since most of these retroperitoneal masses in children are present at birth, this examination is most important in newborns and young infants. The most common retroperitoneal masses are hydronephrosis, caused by improper urinary drainage, and tumors, such as Wilms' tumor and neuroblastoma.

In umbilical hernias it is important to determine the size of the defect in the abdominal wall and not the size of the protruding mass. The examiner checks for inguinal hernias by direct palpation of the inguinal canal and by slipping a finger through the scrotum into the inguinal canal.

In appendicitis, characteristically, there is point tenderness at the junction of the middle two thirds and outer one third of a line drawn between the anterosuperior iliac spine, or anterior tip of the hip bone, and the umbilicus. This is called McBurney's point (see Fig. 5).

Percussion of the abdomen is usually performed to help determine more specifically liver and spleen size and to determine the presence of any abnormal masses. Since the intestine contains more air than solid masses such as spleen, liver, or tumors, the percussion note is resonant over the intestine and becomes dull over these solid masses.

Auscultation of the abdomen will determine presence or absence of bowel sounds as well as increase in bowel sounds. *Bowel sounds* are normal sounds caused by intestinal motility (peristalsis). The examiner must consider all of these findings as a whole in the evaluation of a child. For example, if a child complains of abdominal pain suggestive of appendicitis but has very active bowel sounds, the chances of appendicitis are extremely small (see Chapter 15).

Genitalia. Genitalia are examined by inspection for sexual development, intersex problems, hypospadias, meatal stenosis, presence of testicles, synechia vulva, and normal perforation of the hymen. Digital examination of the genitalia is usually not done before puberty. Should a pelvic examination be necessary before puberty, it is done by rectal examination with the child lying on her side. Synechia vulva, or gluing or sticking together of the labia majora, caused by previous irritation is not an uncommon finding in young girls. It is always important to determine the presence or absence of testicles in boys (see Chapter 16). The examiner must remember that before palpating the testicles it is necessary to close the external inguinal ring at the junction of the scrotum with the abdomen. Closing the external inguinal ring is necessary because children tend to retract their testicles into the inguinal canal when they are afraid, as during a medical examination.

Rectum. Rectal examination is performed on infants at birth to determine whether or not the rectum is open. It is not usually done in routine examinations subsequently, but is done if acute disease such as appendicitis is suspected or if the child has complaints such as anal itching. The rectum is then inspected for irritation and fissures. Fissures are tears in the anus, often caused by constipation.

The examiner must explain to the patient what a rectal examination is in order to calm the patient's fear and enlist his cooperation. The child is then told to lie on his side with his knees flexed. The examiner wears a glove or a finger cot, and a generous amount of lubricant is applied to the gloved finger. The child is told to bear down, just as though he were having a bowel movement. The examiner's finger then touches the rectal sphincter, which will slowly relax. Then the finger is gently introduced into the rectal vault.

Palpation of the rectum by digital examination permits the examiner to determine the tone or tightness of the anal sphincter, the presence or absence of stool in the rectal ampulla, and areas of point tenderness. The tone of the sphincter is lax in neurologic disturbances such as myelomeningocele. The rectal ampulla is full of feces in psychogenic constipation. Although the child may complain when any area is touched, extreme tenderness on the right side is often present with appendicitis.

The rectal examination is the way to do a pelvic examination in young girls. The girl lies on her side and the examiner is able to determine abnormal masses such as retrocecal appendiceal abscess or an ovarian or uterine mass with his finger.

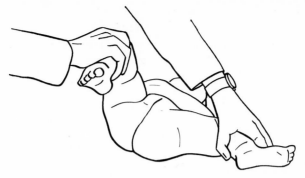

Fig. 6. Maneuver to detect congenital dislocation of the hip.

Extremities. Extremities are examined for deformities, edema, temperature, palmar lines, extra fingers or toes, and pulses, and in the newborn for congenital dislocation of the hip.

Edema is usually determined by pressing on the extremity, usually the lower leg, and watching for a transient depression (pitting).

Palmar lines are often an indication of neurologic and genetic abnormalities. One of the most commonly found abnormal line is a simian line, which is a transverse line in the palm of the hand from one side to the other. It is often seen in Down's syndrome (mongolism).

The usual pulses palpated are the radial and femoral. The radial pulse is well known to nurses and is the most commonly used site to determine pulse rate in children and adults. The femoral pulse is felt in the upper thigh at the junction of the medial one third and outer two thirds. Absence of femoral pulses suggests coarctation of the aorta.

In testing for congenital dislocation of the hip the infant is placed on his back with the thighs flexed. The knees should be capable of passive abduction until they nearly reach the examining table, 70 or more degrees, without resistance. When there is congenital dislocation of the hip, such abduction is possible to only 45 degrees from the perpendicular line established by the vulva or median raphe (see Fig. 6).

Neurologic examination. The neurologic examination can be divided for didactic purposes into three general categories:

1. Examination for meningeal irritation
2. Examination of the newborn
3. Examination of older children

Examination for the presence of meningeal irritation involves observation for paradoxical irritability and performance of specific tests. The term *paradoxical irritability* is used when infants become more upset rather than happier when held. When the infant with meningitis is held his swollen meninges hurt him when he is moved.

Specific indications of meningeal irritation are stiff neck, Kernig's sign, and Brudzinski's sign. When there is meningeal irritation, the patient will resist bending of the neck because it is painful. To elicit Kernig's sign while the patient is lying face up, one bends the thigh at the hip and attempts to extend the leg at the knee. If Kernig's sign is present the patient will resist the latter extension. Brudzinski's sign is sought by bending the neck of a supine patient and noting flexion of the knees. In infants the Brudzinski's sign is more reliable than Kernig's sign.

Neurologic examination in the newborn should include observation of the naked infant to determine alertness, mobility, muscle tone and control, as well as numerous reflexes of which the most important are the *Moro reflex* and the *sucking reflex*. The *Moro reflex* is a normal reflex in infants up to 4 months of age. It is elicited by dropping the baby's head 15 degrees; he then reacts by raising his arms at the shoulders, then flexing his arms at the elbows, clenching his hands, and flexing his knees and hips as if he were grasping a tree; a similar reaction may be elicited by startling the infant. *Sucking reflex* is best evaluated by observing the strength of sucking while feeding the infant. This examination of the newborn will usually tell the examiner not only whether or not the brain responds normally but also whether or not nerves are intact. For example, a newborn who is brain damaged may not have a Moro reflex, and a newborn who has a good brain but has paralysis of the nerve to one arm (brachial paralysis secondary to a traumatic birth) will have a unilateral Moro reflex.

Neurologic examination in older children should include developmental appraisal, evaluation of cranial nerves, evaluation of cerebellar function (balance), and sensory and motor examination. Developmental appraisal is discussed in Chapter 6. A complete neurologic examination including examination of cranial nerves, cerebellar function, and sensory and motor function is one of the most difficult parts of the physical examination. When the nurse practitioner is in doubt she should refer the patient to a competent physician, but before she does so, she should determine gait, muscle control of the eyes, balance, knee jerk reflex, and, in special cases, localized sensory function.

Balance is grossly checked by observation of the gait and by the Romberg test in which the examiner asks the patient to stand with his feet together, his arms extended in a cross, and his eyes closed. The child's ability to stand on one foot is also a useful indication of balance. A 5-year-old child should be able to stand on one foot for 5 seconds (see Chapter 6). Knee jerk, or patella, reflex is tested by tapping the patient with an examining hammer below the knee when the knees are flexed and hanging loosely.

In special cases, such as in a child with a myelomeningocele, the pediatric nurse practitioner should test to see whether or not the child feels pain by pricking him with a pin in order to determine the level of the lesion.

Chapter 4
SCREENING TESTS

Screening tests are part of the routine health supervision. With increasing frequency, paramedical health workers are performing these tests.

The most commonly used screening tests are (1) height and weight, (2) vision and hearing, (3) developmental assessment, (4) urinalysis and hemoglobin, (5) tuberculin test, and (6) biochemical tests (for example, the ferric chloride test for the presence of phenylketonuria and the urinary coproporphyrin test to screen for lead intoxication). Since most of these tests are discussed elsewhere in the text, the present chapter will cover only vision and hearing screening tests.

VISION SCREENING

Vision defects are among the most common handicapping conditions of childhood. Effective screening is of special importance since many of these problems are remediable. Approximately 10 percent of preschool children and 30 percent of school-age children have some kind of impairment of vision. Vision screening tests are valuable because of the high incidence of amblyopia ex anopsia and significant refractive errors. Amblyopia ex anopsia means blindness in one eye caused by lack of use. It occurs when there is enough imbalance, or strabismus, between the two eyes that the child will see double if both eyes are used together. In order not to see double he suppresses vision in one eye without realizing it. The eye in which vision is suppressed becomes almost totally blind from lack of use.

In order to detect excessive heterophoria or latent strabismus the examiner should perform a cover test (Chapter 3). A cover test is done by shining a light 13 to 15 inches in front of the patient's eyes and observing first whether or not the light falls in the center of both pupils. One eye is then covered with a card, which is quickly removed so that the examiner may observe any eye movement. In case of suspected latent strabismus, the child should be referred to an ophthalmologist.

The Snellen chart with letters of different sizes is used to measure visual acuity of children who have learned the alphabet. First both eyes are tested together and then each eye is tested individually. If vision in either eye is less than 20/40, the patient should be referred to an ophthalmologist. From approximately 3 years of age to the time when the child knows the alphabet other vision screening tests can be used, one of the most common of which is the Snellen Illiterate E test. The Snellen Illiterate E is similar to the Snellen chart but is useful for children before they learn the alphabet, since the child is simply asked to indicate which direction the three legs of the letter "E" are pointing. If visual acuity is less than 20/40 in either eye, the child should be referred to an ophthalmologist.

HEARING SCREENING

Most available screening tests detect hearing impairment in 10 percent of infants and 3 percent of school-age children. These hearing screening tests depend on mechanical devices which produce either pure tones of different frequencies at different decibels of intensity (pure tone audiometry) or human voice at different intensity (speech audiometry).

Pure tone air conduction audiometry is a commonly used test for hearing screening. It can be performed in both ears simultaneously and in groups of children; however, whenever possible, hearing screening should be done individually and monaurally. For the purpose of screening, the intensity is usually set at 20 decibels if the room is noise-free and 30 decibels in noisy rooms. Frequencies of 500, 2,000 and 4,000 cycles per second are utilized, since most human speech is within this range.

Chronic serous otitis media, which will be discussed in Chapter 12, is a significant treatable factor producing hearing impairment. Impaction of cerumen is also a common cause of hearing deficit. Damage to the auditory nerve due to diseases such as mumps may also produce hearing impairment.

Chapter 5
GROWTH AND DEVELOPMENT

Knowledge of growth and development is of extreme importance in evaluating children, since chronically ill children do not grow well.

Growth, which means increase in size, and *development,* which means increase in skill and complexity of function, depend on heredity as well as on intrauterine and extrauterine conditions.

The *prenatal period* is the period from conception to the day of birth, which is usually around the 280th day of gestation. An *embryo* is the unborn child from conception to nine weeks of gestation. The fetus is the unborn child from nine weeks to birth. The *newborn* period includes the first 4 weeks of extrauterine life. *Infancy* is the first year of life. *Preschool years,* or early childhood, cover the period from 1 to 6 years of age. *Prepubertal stage,* or late childhood, is from 6 years to the beginning of adolescence, at about 10 years of age. *Adolescence* starts with acceleration of growth in height and weight, is followed by the appearance of secondary sex characteristics and deceleration of growth, and terminates with the union of the epiphyses, cessation of linear growth, and the development of the ability to reproduce. *Puberty* refers to the time of appearance of dark pigmented pubic hair.

HEREDITY

Heredity is the result of the differences among the genes that determine the physical and biochemical characteristics of each individual. *Genes* are the smallest units determining heredity. They are arranged in groups in a linear fashion; each group is called a *chromosome.* Each person has 22 pairs of chromosomes called autosomes and one additional pair which determines sex, the sex chromosomes. Therefore, there are a total of 46 chromosomes in the normal person. *Karyotyping* is the process of mapping or identifying the chromosomes. There are numerous genetic clinical syndromes that are associated with abnormalities of chromosomes, such as mongolism, or Down's syndrome, in which there are 47 chromosomes and Turner's syndrome in which there are 45 chromosomes with absence of one sex chromosome.

Most hereditary diseases are due to characteristics of a single gene or pair of genes. When only one of the pair of genes transmits a disease, the gene is dominant; when both genes of a pair are required to transmit the disease, the gene is recessive. When a disease is transmitted through a dominant gene, an affected person will have a 50 percent chance of transmitting the disease to his progeny if the marital partner is not affected. In diseases transmitted through a recessive gene, such as sickle cell anemia, the result of the union of two unaffected individuals who are "carriers" of the gene will be: 25 percent of the progeny will be normal, 50 percent will be carriers, and 25 percent will have the disease. Other diseases such as hemophilia are linked to the sex chromosomes.

When a hereditary disease or trait is identified, genetic counseling should be offered to the parents.

PLACENTA

The placenta is an organ of utmost importance for the development of the unborn child, since it functions as his lung, kidney, and gastrointestinal tract.

The placenta functions as the unborn child's lungs since blood oxygenation occurs across the placenta. It functions as the child's kidneys since the child disposes of waste products across the placenta. It functions as the child's gastrointestinal tract, since the child obtains nutrients from his mother through the placenta.

Placental dysfunction at or near delivery results in death or signs of fetal distress caused by anoxia. Placental dysfunction of lesser degree can occur throughout pregnancy and results in a "malnourished" infant who is small for his gestational age at birth.

BIRTH WEIGHT

The birth weight of 2,500 grams (5 pounds 8 ounces), is used to separate low birth weight infants from other newborns.

Low birth weight infants have more problems (congenital anomalies, mental retardation, and neurologic abnormalities) than newborns of normal birth weight.

Low birth weight may be the result of prematurity or intrauterine growth retardation. Different problems are associated with each of these conditions. For example, the neonatal death rate of premature infants is higher than for full-term infants because of the respiratory distress syndrome. Infants with intrauterine growth retardation tend to show failure to thrive. Infants in categories of low birth weight have a significantly higher number of problems than normal newborns.

Infants of diabetic or prediabetic mothers, although large for their individual gestational age, also have a higher risk of neonatal problems, especially respiratory distress syndrome and hypoglycemia.

MEASUREMENTS

A child should be compared with his peers in order to determine whether his growth rate is appropriate or not. Chronically ill children do not grow well.

The two most common ways to compare a child with his peers are through the use of a percentile chart or a mean standard deviation chart. Weight, height, and infants' head circumference are the measurements most frequently utilized. A percentile chart shows the distribution of measurements in a typical series of 100 children. Thus, the tenth percentile gives the value for the tenth child of a group of 100; that is, nine children will be smaller and ninety will be larger in the measurement under consideration. Each individual child will tend to grow along a given pattern. Usually a child who falls in the tenth percentile for height at 6 months of age will be near the tenth percentile at 2 years. Marked changes in percentiles, either increases or decreases, may indicate disease.

A mean standard deviation chart is based on the mean (the arithmetic average) of a particular measurement at a particular age. Variability around the mean is expressed in standard deviations. One standard deviation includes 66 percent of the observations, two standard deviations include 95 percent of the observations, and three standard deviations include 99 percent of the observations. Therefore, a measurement at three standard deviations above the mean indicates that 99 percent of the child's peers will have measurements smaller than that particular measurement; a measurement 3 standard deviations below the mean indicates that 99 percent of the child's peers will have measurements larger than that particular measurement.

Head. Head growth is of utmost importance during the first year of life since one half of the growth in head size occurs in this period. During the first year of life the head grows 4 inches in circumference; it then grows 2 inches from 1 to 7 years, and 2 inches from 7 to 20 years.

Height and weight. Rates of weight gain and height increments are significantly different; for example, there is a relative decrease in weight gain between ages 2 and 3 years when the child loses his baby fat as compared to the rate of linear growth in that period. There is a relative increase in weight during the prepubertal years producing some chubbiness between ages 9 to 11 years because the rate of weight gain is faster than the rate of linear growth during that period. Birth weight is usually doubled by the fourth month of life and tripled by 1 year. On the other hand, birth length is not doubled until age 4 years and not tripled until age 12.

Some useful rules of thumb regarding height and weight are as follows:

Weight first year of life

Age in months + 11 = weight in pounds

Weight 1 year to puberty

(5 × age in years) + 18 = weight in pounds

Height 2 to 14 years

(2 × age in years) + 32 = height in inches

TEETH

The average baby gets his first tooth at about 7 months, but he has been drooling, biting, and having crying periods from the age of 3 or 4 months as a prelude to that first tooth. Since the first dentition consists of 20 teeth and they all come between 7 months and 2½ years of age it is easy to see why babies are teething most of their first 2½ years.

Usually the first two teeth to erupt are the lower central incisors; these are followed by the four upper incisors, which erupt by 1 year of age. At about 14 months the first molars appear followed by the cuspids (canines) by 18 months and the second molars by 2 years of age.

Permanent teeth usually start to erupt at 7 years of age. The first permanent teeth to appear are the central lower incisors and the first molar behind the primary teeth. The rest of the incisors, cuspids, and bicuspids appear between the ages of 8 and 11 years. These are followed by the 12-year molars (second molar) and finally by the wisdom teeth (third molar) at 18 years.

BLOOD

During the first 3 months, because of several not-well-understood reasons, the bone marrow is relatively inactive and the rate of body growth is very fast. Hemoglobin goes from about 18 grams per 100 ml at birth to 10 grams per 100 ml at 3 months. This is called physiologic anemia.

At the lowest point of physiologic anemia, at about 3 months of age, the bone marrow starts working faster and iron begins to be utilized in a significant fashion. Babies born at term have enough iron reserve to last them until age 6 months, and as long as there is establishment of dietary iron intake the infant does not develop iron deficiency anemia. If the infant continues on an iron deficient diet (milk alone), he will develop iron deficiency anemia by age 9 to 18 months.

The baby born prematurely goes through the same cycle, but the first postnatal decrease of hemoglobin occurs early and usually reaches lower levels. This anemia is, therefore, called anemia of prematurity, rather than physiologic anemia. Premature infants require additional medicinal iron, since they are born with less iron reserve than term babies and since anemia of prematurity occurs earlier and is more severe than physiologic anemia. However, although iron is required to produce hemoglobin in premature infants after 2 to 3 months of age, it neither prevents nor helps anemia of prematurity, but it does prevent iron deficiency anemia that often occurs at the end of the first year in premature infants.

BONE

Development of osseous epiphyseal centers occurs in a certain order with specific centers appearing at specific ages. This skeletal maturation can be detected by x-rays so that a radiologist is able to determine bone age, which is a useful tool in evaluating children with growth disorders. Most commonly the epiphyseal centers of the wrists and hands are used to determine bone age after 3 months of age; in newborn infants the knees are used.

Chapter 6
DEVELOPMENTAL APPRAISAL

In evaluating central nervous system development or level of maturation the nurse practitioner must consider neuromuscular development, behavior, and personality development. Developmental screening tests and psychometric testing are useful tools for evaluating this important aspect of health.

NEUROMUSCULAR DEVELOPMENT

Neuromuscular developmental progress during the first year of life occurs in a cephalocaudal and proximodistal direction; that is, it goes from control of the eyes and head during the first quarter of the first year to integration of the legs in the erect posture at the end of the first year. The pediatric nurse practitioner should know some significant milestones in neuromuscular development of children in order to take a good developmental history. Table 2 shows some important developmental milestones during the first 5 years of life. In older children performance in school becomes important, and in some situations makes it unnecessary to obtain an early developmental history; however, in other circumstances, as in school underachievement, early developmental milestones are important. For example, it is unimportant to obtain a good early developmental history on an adolescent who is well-adjusted and is doing well in school. On the other hand, if the same adolescent is not achieving normally in school, both early developmental history and some indications of the child's interpersonal relationships become significant.

Furthermore, it is well to stress that although these developmental milestones are asked in the history and noted during the physical examination, the order of occurrence is not absolute, and considerable variation does occur. For example, many children pull up and walk without crawling and many toddlers do not walk until 15 months of age. A similar range of variation will be noted throughout life and is noted in the Denver Developmental Scale by indicating the percent of normal children who carry out a particular function at a given age (see fold-out).

Table 2. Developmental milestones

At 1 month the child regards an object
At 2 months the child smiles
At 3 months the child turns his head
At 4 months the child holds his head
At 5 months the child rolls over
At 6 months the child transfers objects
At 7 months the child sits briefly
At 8 months the child creeps
At 9 months the child pulls up
At 10 months the child walks with support
At 11 months the child stands alone
At 12 months the child walks alone and uses 2 to 3 words
At 2 years the child uses 3 word sentences
At 3 years the child draws a circle and rides a tricycle
At 4 years the child draws a square
At 5 years the child draws a triangle, ties shoes, and buttons buttons

BEHAVIOR

Behavior, although indivisible, can crudely but usefully be separated for clinical use into five major areas: gross motor, fine motor, language, personal-social, and adaptive.

Gross motor behavior includes control of the head, trunk, and extremities. Fine motor development pertains to the achievement of control of fine movements of the fingers. Motor behavior is important in evaluating neurologic integrity. Although motor behavior gives some indication of intellectual development, it is important to avoid the mistake of using acquisitions of motor control as the sole criterion of intellectual ability.

Language may be divided into two areas: receptive and expressive. Expressive language includes the production of sound, single words, and combination of words as well as nonverbal expressions for the purpose of communication. Receptive language includes response to sounds and speech and the understanding of words. Although language is useful in evaluating intellectual development, it may be incorrectly used as the only criterion of intelligence.

The personal-social aspect of behavior has the widest variation of all fields, since it includes the individual's knowledge and acceptance of himself as well as his adequate integration in society. Although dependent to a large extent on culture and environment, its expression is also a function of neuromotor maturity.

Adaptive behavior includes manipulation or exploration of objects, the use of motor capacities in the execution of practical tasks, and the utilization of past experiences in the solution of new problems. Adaptive behavior is the area of behavior most commonly assessed when measuring intellectual potential.

DEVELOPMENTAL SCREENING TESTS

Somewhat more specific than using the history of developmental milestones is to use one of the accepted developmental scales. One of the most commonly used in the first 6 years of life, because of its reliability and ease of administration, is the Denver Developmental Scale. Instructions for the use of the Denver Developmental Scale can be obtained from LADOCA Project and Publishing Foundation, Inc., Denver, Colorado (see fold-out). Another developmental test that is useful after age 3 is the Goodenough Draw-A-Person test, in which the child is asked to draw a person; specific criteria are provided to evaluate his drawing. The child may also simply be asked to draw geometric figures; his level of neurologic maturation and intellectual functioning will influence his ability to draw these figures (see Table 2).

There are also other more verbal tests such as, the Kent Emergency Scale and Ammon Quick Test, to determine intellectual development in older children. The former can be obtained from the Psychological Corporation in New York City and the latter from the Psychological Test Specialist in Missoula, Montana. A nurse practitioner may need to administer these simple tests in screening for intelligence, especially if there is question about the patient's intellectual performance.

PSYCHOMETRIC TESTS

Whenever it is suspected, after developmental screening testing, that a child has an intellectual deficiency, a psychometric test to measure intelligence by a psychologist becomes mandatory.

In psychometric tests such as the Infant Cattell, Bayley Scale, Stanford-Binet, or Wechsler Intelligence Scale, intelligence is expressed comparatively as a score derived by dividing the child's mental age (MA) obtained in the test by the chronologic age (CA) and multiplying the result by 100. This number is referred to as the intelligence quotient (IQ). It should always be remembered that psychometric testing can be inaccurate, since it represents only a specific sampling of the child's ability to perform at a specific time in a specific situation.

An experienced psychologist will always evaluate the probable validity of the test results by noting the child's behavior during the testing session, degree of anxiety, interest in task provided, and eagerness of performance.

PERSONALITY DEVELOPMENT

There are two major general approaches in the evaluation of personality development: (1) the psychoanalytic theory and (2) the behaviorist theory. Neither one has been universally accepted and both are useful tools in the treatment of behavior problems.

The *psychoanalytic theory* views the personality as formed by three parts: id (instinct), ego (mediator between instinctual drives and the outer world), and superego (censor concerning acceptability of thoughts, feelings, and behavior). According to psychoanalytic theory, there are two main instinctual drives—sexual instinct and aggressive instinct. Children are said to pass through five stages of psychosexual development which are: *oral phase* (0 to 1 year), *anal phase* (1 to 3 years) *phallic phase* (3 to 6 years), *latency* (6 to 12 years), and *adolescence.* In each of these phases there are ways to gratify instincts and there are also specific ego defense mechanisms and superego censorship. The Oedipus complex or feeling in the child—a tendency to possessiveness toward the parent of the opposite sex and rivalry toward the parent of the same sex—is very centrally located in psychosexual development. Inability to properly pass through the different phases of psychosexual development produces emotional arrests which, according to psychoanalytic theory, are the basis of mental illness.

Those following *behavioristic theory* of personality do not seek reasons for specific behavior in the person's past, but rather look at the expression of problems or symptoms and try to correct them by operant conditioning. In operant conditioning the environment is programmed to respond to the subject's behavior with planned rewards for the desired act. For example, in utilizing positive reinforcement in treating enuresis the operant behaviorist would reward the child with specific rewards every morning that he wakes up dry, without looking for possible causes of the enuresis in the patient's personal and family situations, as a psychoanalytic therapist would do.

Chapter 7

LABORATORY PROCEDURES

The complete evaluation of a patient often includes several laboratory procedures. In some situations pediatric nurse practitioners will perform these procedures directly; in other situations they will delegate the responsibility to community health workers.

BLOOD

In ambulatory pediatrics the most important tests in the examination of the blood are hemoglobin and hematocrit determinations and white blood cell and differential counts.

Hemoglobin and hematocrit. Hemoglobin or hematocrit determination are part of health supervision and are of extreme importance in the detection of anemia, especially at the end of the first year of life when nutritional iron deficiency anemia is often present.

Hemoglobin is measured in grams per 100 milliliters of blood, and hematocrit is measured in percent of volume of red cells contained in whole blood after centrifugations.

Methods to determine hemoglobin concentrations are *visual,* such as the Sahli or the Spencer-Hb-Meter of the American Optical Company, and *photoelectric* methods, which require more expensive equipment. Hematocrit values depend only on centrifugation of the blood and are, therefore, more reliable in experienced hands.

The normal hemoglobin changes during the first year of life are discussed in Chapter 5. After the first year of life any child with hemoglobin below 11 grams per 100 ml is anemic.

Although anemia by definition is a decrease in hemoglobin, the hematocrit has the advantage, as stated above, of being less subject to technical errors and having a relatively fixed relationship with the hemoglobin. Hematocrits, in volumes percent, correspond to three times the concentrations of hemoglobin in grams per 100 ml. For example, a hematocrit of 30 percent corresponds to a hemoglobin value of 10 grams per 100 ml.

White blood cell count. The white blood cell count is of importance in evaluating children with acute illnesses, since it varies with many diseases and thus helps to determine both the severity of the illness and its possible etiology.

A white blood cell count measures the number of white cells per cubic millimeter of blood by either photoelectric or visual techniques. In visual methods the blood is diluted 1 to 20 with hydrochloric or acetic acid in a special pipette, and the cells in the four large peripheral squares of a Neubauer counting chamber are counted.

Normally the white blood cell count is 5,000 to 10,000 per cubic millimeter of blood. It is generally normal or decreased in some viral infections, such as rubella and rubeola, and elevated in bacterial infections such as streptococcal pharyngitis. The white blood cell count can be normally elevated during the first 2 weeks of life and interpretation of the significance of a specific count during this period of life is almost impossible unless the count is very depressed (below 5,000 cells per cubic millimeter). A depressed white blood cell count in the presence of a bacterial infection, both in newborn and older children, may indicate overwhelming infection to which the patient's defense mechanism is unable to respond.

Differential white blood cell count. The differential white blood cell count shows the relative number of the different types of white cells. It is also useful in evaluating children with acute illnesses, since it sheds light on the nature and severity of the illness.

A thin blood smear is made and stained with a differential stain such as Wright or Leishman stain; 100 white cells are then counted under the microscope to determine the percentage of each type of cell present (lymphocytes, monocytes, and granulocytes—neutrophils, eosinophils, and basophils).

Normally, lymphocytes and neutrophils account for approximately 90 percent of the white blood cells. There is a predominance of lymphocytes (40 to 60 percent) up to 6 years of age, after which there is a predominance of granulocytes, mostly neutrophils (40 to 60 percent). Pathologic or disease states alter the differential white blood cell count. The classical examples are bacterial infections, in which there is usually an increase of neutrophils, and allergic parasitic disease, in which there is an increase of eosinophils above its normal value of 1 to 3 percent.

URINE

A urinalysis is indicated at several specific scheduled intervals during routine health supervision as well as when urinary tract disease is suspected by the symptomatology (see Chapters 10 and 16).

A routine urinalysis covers three major areas: inspection, chemical examination, and microscopic examination.

Inspection is simple observation of the urine specimen for color and transparency. Color may be yellow, tea-colored, bloody, and so on, and the degree of transparency may range from clear to cloudy.

Chemical examination has become extremely simple with the development of quick methods of detecting significant aspects of the chemical composition of the urine and the presence of abnormal chemical elements. One of the most complete and easy to use chemical methods is the Labstix method. A strip of plastic tagged with different reagents is dipped into the urine specimen and produces a colorimetric reaction indicating urinary pH and the presence of protein, glucose, ketones, and blood. Ferric chloride examination for phenylketonuria will be discussed later in this chapter.

Microscopic examination of the urine consists of examining under the microscope a drop of urine or its sediment after 10 ml have been spun in a centrifuge for 5 to 10 minutes. The examiner looks both for bacteria, which, if present, are usually motile, rod-like organisms, and for formed elements (white blood cells, red blood cells, and casts).

Normally the urine is clear and yellow and does not contain protein, glucose, ketones, or blood as measured by screening chemical methods.

A tea-colored urine may indicate hepatitis or the presence of degraded blood; a cloudy "smoky" urine may indicate hematuria as seen in glomerulonephritis. Abnormal amounts of protein in the urine may suggest urinary tract infection, nephrosis, or glomerulonephritis. Glucose in the urine may indicate diabetes mellitus.

Microscopic examination of a drop of urine should reveal no red cells and only an occasional white blood cell. When the urine is spun, examination of the wet sediment should reveal no red blood cells; however, white blood cells may normally be as numerous as 0 to 3 per high power field, and an occasional hyaline cast may be also found. The presence of rod-shaped bacteria in a drop of fresh, properly collected unspun urine indicates urinary tract infection.

Ideally, urinalysis, especially microscopic examination, should be done on fresh, midstream, clean catch urine; this is most important in older girls in whom vaginal secretions contain white blood cells and bacteria. Bacteria multiply readily and cells and casts may be destroyed when urine is allowed to stand at room temperature. In consequence, the urine should be examined as soon as possible.

Ferric chloride test. Ferric chloride is a chemical test of importance in newborns and young infants to determine the presence or absence of abnormal products indicative of phenylketonuria, which is a disease that causes mental retardation.

One or two drops of 10 percent ferric chloride are overlayed on 1 ml of urine. If a urine specimen is unavailable, a drop of urine on a wet diaper may be tested. The development of a green color of the urine may indicate the presence of abnormal products that are found in phenylketonuria and should prompt further investigation.

In some states a ferric chloride test is mandatory by law in all newborns; in others a Guthrie blood test is required. The *Guthrie test* checks for a specific bacterial growth that requires phenylalanine for its metabolism.

STOOL

The nurse practitioner needs familiarity with examination of the stool for pH as well as for white blood or "pus" cells and parasitic eggs.

Stool pH is measured by dipping nitrazine paper into the stool and comparing the reaction with a color chart; an acid pH indicates the presence of malabsorption due to disaccharidase intolerance. Temporary disaccharidase intolerance often occurs after an acute episode of diarrhea.

Parasite eggs, except for pinworm eggs and pus cells, can be found in the stool by placing a drop of saline on a slide and adding stool with an applicator until the drop in the slide becomes cloudy. The slide is then examined under the microscope. Pus cells in the stool are usually indicative of bacterial infection.

Pinworms are the most widespread parasite in the United States today; the eggs, and at times the entire worm, are found by blotting around the anus with the adhesive side of clear tape, placing the tape on a glass slide, and looking at it under a microscope. The patient's parents are often asked to prepare the tape when the child first wakes up, since pinworms tend to come out to lay eggs more often at night. Pinworms are thin, motile, white worms measuring between 3 and 13 mm. The eggs are ovoid and contain a larva inside.

CEREBROSPINAL FLUID

Examination of cerebrospinal fluid is an absolute necessity in patients with suspected meningitis. Pediatric nurse practitioners should not examine cerebrospinal fluid by themselves; however, they need to know the significance of cerebrospinal fluid findings.

The fluid should be examined by inspection for color and clarity; chemically for sugar and protein content, which is done by the laboratory; and microscopically directly and after the addition of acetic acid to lyse the red blood cells. Bacteriologic cultures are important, and these are done by the laboratory.

Normally the cerebrospinal fluid is colorless and transparent, its sugar content is one half to two thirds that of the blood, its protein content is less than 40 mg per 100 ml, and its cell content is up to eight mononuclear cells per cubic millimeter. In bacterial meningitis the fluid is usually cloudy with decreased sugar and elevated protein levels, and an increased number of cells, often more than 100 per cubic millimeter.

CULTURES

Accurate diagnosis in infectious diseases depends upon obtaining the right culture from the right secretion or body fluid in the right way, as well as on adequate processing of the specimen in the laboratory.

The pediatric nurse practitioner needs to know how to obtain, incubate, and read throat cultures for group A beta hemolytic streptococcus, since they are commonly used ambulatory procedures. Early detection and treatment of streptococcal disease prevents rheumatic fever.

The examiner obtains a throat culture by swabbing the throat with a cotton-tipped applicator and subsequently touching the applicator to a blood agar plate, which is then streaked with a wire loop and incubated overnight at 37° C.

Group A beta hemolytic streptococci colonies are small white colonies surrounded by a zone of beta hemolysis of blood—a clear zone—in the blood agar plate.

GRAM STAIN

The gram stain is a stain for bacteria and is based on the ability of bacteria to become stained by crystal violet.

A drop of fluid suspected of containing bacteria, such as pus, sputum, and sometimes urine, is air dried and gently heat fixed on a slide. The slide is stained with crystal violet, which is blue, and then with a red dye (safranine) for contrast.

Bacteria such as streptococcus, staphylococcus, or pneumoccocus are designated gram positive because they take the blue crystal violet; gram negative bacteria, such as hemophilus influenza, do not. These staining characteristics are important because bacterial sensitivity to antibiotic medications is frequently associated with their staining characteristics by this technique (see Chapter 22).

Chapter 8
IMMUNIZATIONS

Immunization is the most specific tool a practitioner of medicine has to prevent illnesses. At the present time, the immunizations most frequently used are against the following diseases: diphtheria, pertussis, tetanus, poliomyelitis, smallpox, rubeola, rubella and mumps. Although each clinic or physician's office uses a specific immunization schedule, most schedules follow the recommendations of the Committee on Infectious Diseases of the American Academy of Pediatrics.

IMMUNIZING AGENTS

Immunizing agents are antigens (see Chapter 13). Some are nonviable. These are either dead organisms or modified products of organisms (toxoid). Nonviable vaccines include diphtheria, tetanus, pertussis, and Salk poliomyelitis vaccines. Other vaccines are live or attenuated live organisms, such as Sabin poliomyelitis vaccine, smallpox, rubella, and the most commonly used rubeola vaccine.

With nonviable vaccines the antibody response is due entirely to the antigenic dosage, which can be very high; with vaccines of living organisms antibody production depends on viral multiplication in the host receiving the vaccine.

Vaccines of nonviable organisms or toxoids have been combined as with diphtheria, pertussis, and tetanus. More recently combinations of live virus vaccines have been given experimentally. Combinations of live viruses were not recommended in the past; however, the current Committee on Infectious Diseases of the American Academy of Pediatrics feels that simultaneous administration of various live virus vaccines is acceptable. It is felt that the theoretical fear of production of viral interference has been overweighed by the lack of evidence of real interference and by the practicality of decreasing the number of necessary visits to the health facility.

Diphtheria-pertussis-tetanus (DPT). Diphtheria-pertussis-tetanus (DPT) is usually given to children below 6 years of age. Each antigen can be given separately but it is more convenient to give them together, and, according to some sources, the combination of the three antigens together with an adjuvant (a triple depot aluminum precipitated antigen) probably produces a better immunity.

After the age of 6 years the risk of complications from pertussis is diminished and the risk of a vaccine-induced convulsion increases. Therefore, pertussis vaccine is not recommended for children over 6 years of age. Since the chances of reaction to diphtheria vaccine are greater in older children "adult type" of combined diphtheria and tetanus vaccines (Adult dT), which contains a lesser concentration of diphtheria vaccine, should be given after age 6.

Poliomyelitis. The two major types of poliomyelitis vaccines are the killed virus vaccine developed by Salk and the live attenuated virus vaccine developed by Sabin. The former is administered intramusculary and the latter orally (OPV). With increasing frequency live attenuated virus is used because it produces much better immunity with minimal possibility of reaction, and it is easier to administer.

If the primary series of live attenuated poliomyelitis vaccine is administered after the first birthday no further recall immunizations are required in areas where poliomyelitis is nonprevalent. If the vaccine is given to infants (see Table 3) further "boosters" are required at ages 15 to 18 months and 4 to 6 years because of interference by maternal antibodies. Live attenuated poliomyelitis vaccine should not be given to breast-fed infants until after weaning, since poliomyelitis antibodies transferred through the milk prevent virus multiplication and the development of immunity.

Smallpox. Smallpox vaccine is a live virus vaccine. In a classic "primary take" a small red papule surrounded by reddish skin will appear within 3 to 5 days. This papule will soon become a blister and by 10 to 12 days, a scab will form. This scab will get dark and fall in 3 to 4 weeks. Smallpox vaccine should not be given to children having skin rashes or to children with siblings having skin rashes because of the possibility of generalized spread, a condition called eczema vaccinatum.

Since children under 1 year of age and older than 2 years have a slightly higher incidence of complications—either generalized spread through broken skin or postvaccination encephalitis—the vaccine should be administered for the first time (primary immunization) to children between 1 and 2 years of age.

Rubeola. Rubeola (hard measles) vaccine is a live attenuated virus vaccine. A few children develop fever and a rash 7 to 10 days after its administration, and parents should be warned regarding this possibility. As in the case of live poliomyelitis vaccine viral multiplication is essential and therefore the vaccine should be administered after the first year of life, when maternally acquired antibodies will not interfere with viral multiplication.

Rubella. Rubella (German or three-day measles) vaccine is also a live attenuated virus vaccine. Joint pain and arthritis are rare complications following its administration. This reaction may occur even 4 to 6 weeks after administration of the vaccine and is most common in adults and older children. The rubella vaccine should be given after the first year of life

Table 3. Immunization schedule of the American Academy of Pediatrics*

2 months	DPT-trivalent OPV
3 months	DPT
4 months	DPT-trivalent OPV
6 months	Trivalent OPV
12 months	Tuberculin test followed by live attenuated measles, at the time of reading the tuberculin test if test is negative; tuberculin yearly thereafter
15-18 months	DPT-trivalent OPV-Smallpox
4-6 years	DPT-trivalent OPV-Smallpox
12-14 years	dT-Smallpox-Mumps

Thereafter dT every 10 years; smallpox every 3 to 10 years

Rubella—before puberty in females to be sure they are not pregnant, since the vaccine is contraindicated in pregnancy

*From Report of the Committee on Infectious Diseases, 1970, American Academy of Pediatrics, page 5.

because of the possibility of maternal antibodies interfering with viral multiplication.

Mumps. Mumps vaccine is a live attenuated viral vaccine. Since mumps is essentially a benign disease during childhood, the vaccine at present is recommended only for nonimmune children immediately before puberty. This recommendation may change when more experience is gained with the vaccine, particularly regarding the duration of immunity.

Tuberculin test. Although tuberculin is not a vaccine, it is discussed in this chapter because it is a diagnostic test that is included in most immunization schedules for health supervision (see Table 3).

Tuberculin testing depends on cellular immunity (see Chapter 13) and, if positive, indicates that the patient has or has had contact with the organisms that produce tuberculosis *(Mycobacterium tuberculosis)*. The pediatric nurse practitioner should be aware of the fact that the antituberculosis vaccine, BCG, which is widely administered in many countries and in specific areas of the United States to high risk children, may also produce a positive tuberculin test. Therefore, a positive tuberculin test is not exclusively an indication of contact with virulent tuberculosis organism, since it may be the result of previous immunization with the antituberculosis vaccine.

Tuberculin testing depends on the intradermal injection of dead tuberculosis bacilli (old tuberculin) or the introduction of a filtrate of tuberculosis bacilli cultures, such as the so-called purified protein derivative (PPD).

A dose of old tuberculin (OT) and purified protein derivative (PPD) may contain 1, 5, 10, or between 100 and 250 tuberculin units depending on the dilution. A reaction of 10 mm induration 48 to 72 hours after the intradermal introduction of 5 to 10 tuberculin units is considered a positive tuberculin reaction. Reactions between 5 and 10 mm of induration are doubtful, and the patient needs further evaluation.

For screening purposes the Heaf multiple puncture test with the sterneedle "gun" and special glycerinated PPD and the Tine test, which consists of a stainless steel disk with four prongs precoated with OT, are gaining wide acceptance. Induration of one or more of the puncture sites of 2 mm or more in diameter is considered positive. The child should be observed for reaction after 3 days; however, the Heaf test should be observed for reaction up to 1 week.

IMMUNIZATION SCHEDULE

The present schedule of immunizations recommended by the American Academy of Pediatrics is shown in Table 3.

CONTRAINDICATIONS

Before beginning immunizations, the pediatric nurse practitioner should be aware of certain contraindications. The presence of an acute illness, a previously severe reaction to the same vaccine, the presence of skin rashes, pregnancy, malignancies, or compromised immunologic response are situations that need careful consideration before immunizations are given.

When a child has an acute febrile illness, such as an upper respiratory infection, immunization should be deferred.

If any antigen has previously produced a severe reaction (such as fever above 103° F, somnolence, or convulsion), the subsequent dose should be given with caution and should be smaller than the standard dose. In many cases subsequent doses should consist of single antigens and a specific antigen may need to be omitted; for example, with diphtheria-tetanus-pertussis vaccine, pertussis produces reactions most often and is the antigen most commonly deleted in subsequent doses.

The presence of skin rash (eczema) in a patient or a sibling is a contraindication to smallpox vaccination because the vaccine may spread through the areas of broken skin producing eczema vaccinatum, which is often fatal.

Rubella vaccine is contraindicated during pregnancy. Live virus vaccines are contraindicated in patients with malignancies or compromised immunologic response.

The pediatric nurse practitioner also needs to remember that since tuberculosis tends to spread in the presence of measles, the measles vaccine is never given to patients who have active tuberculosis. Thus, tuberculin testing is mandatory before the administration of live measles vaccine.

Chapter 9

NUTRITION

Because children must have proper nutrition for optimal growth and development, nutritional knowledge becomes fundamental for persons responsible for health supervision in pediatrics. Supplying only the caloric requirements is not sufficient to promote optimal growth. Each of the basic foodstuffs —water, protein, carbohydrates, fat, minerals, and vitamins—must be considered quantitatively and individually.

CALORIC REQUIREMENTS

Children, in order to have energy for optimal growth, should be provided with calories to allow for: (1) basal metabolism (maintenance of body function at rest), (2) specific dynamic action of foods (increase over basal metabolism brought about by ingestion and assimilation of food), (3) growth, (4) muscular activity, and (5) caloric loss in excreta. Basal caloric requirements gradually decrease from about 55 calories per kilogram of body weight per day in infants to 25 to 30 calories per kilogram of body weight per 24 hours in adults.

Specific dynamic action (SDA) of food is about 5 to 7 calories per kilogram of body weight per day in most general diets. The unused caloric loss in stool is about 10 percent of the daily intake.

Requirements for growth and muscular activity, as expected, vary tremendously for specific individuals at different age levels at different times and for the two sexes. For example, a 14-year-old in training for football will require many more calories than a 14-year-old boy who is not in training.

BASIC FOODSTUFFS

Water. Water is second only to oxygen as an essential for existence. Water constitutes 70 percent of the body weight of an infant and 60 percent of an adult. Since requirements for water are related to caloric expenditure, infants require larger volumes per body weight than adults. Infants become dehydrated more readily when deprived of water or when they lose excessive water, as with diarrhea.

Proteins. Proteins are the predominant solid structure of the body. They are formed by amino acids. There are nine amino acids essential for children and eight that are essential for adults. They must be ingested because the human body cannot synthesize them from other foodstuffs. Good dietary sources of proteins are milk, eggs, meat, fish, poultry, cheese, soybeans, peas, beans, and nuts.

Carbohydrates. Carbohydrates provide the greatest portion of the caloric needs. They also are the most readily available source of energy. Good dietary sources of carbohydrates are milk, cereal, fruits, syrup, starches, and vegetables.

Fats. Fats are the most concentrated source of energy. They also spare protein and are important for the synthesis of steroid hormones. Fats are formed by fatty acids, two of which, linoleic acid and arachidonic acid are essential. Good dietary sources of fats are milk, butter, egg yolk, lard, bacon, meat, cheese, nuts, and vegetable oil.

Minerals. Minerals are essential to the body structure and function. The principal minerals of physiologic importance are calcium, chloride, cobalt, fluoride, iodide, magnesium, potassium, sodium, phosphorus, and sulfur. The diet should be supplemented with fluoride if the water supply does not contain an adequate content. Otherwise, an unrestricted diet that includes milk usually provides adequate amounts of minerals.

Vitamins. Vitamins are organic compounds that are required in minute amounts for energy and cellular metabolism. They are therefore essential for maintenance and growth of the organism. The essential vitamins (A, B complex, C, D, and E) are usually consumed in an unrestricted diet. Vitamin K is synthesized by intestinal bacteria.

In most areas in the United States milk is supplemented with vitamins A and D and cereals and bread are supplemented with some of the B vitamins, particularly pyridoxine and thiamine. Infants need medicinal supplementation of vitamins C and D until 2 years of age. Commercially prepared infant formulas have added vitamins, including vitamins C and D. After age 2, children consuming a balanced diet receive their daily vitamin requirements through natural food sources. In some disorders, however, the fat-soluble vitamins A, D, and to some extent K, are poorly absorbed and special water-soluble preparations need to be given. This is true in malabsorption syndromes such as cystic fibrosis of the pancreas and in patients with obstructive liver disease in whom fats are poorly absorbed.

In many countries where there is no vitamin supplementation of food, vitamin deficiencies are frequent.

APPETITE

Mothers of children between 18 and 36 months of age often complain about their children's poor appetite. "My 2-year-old Johnny does not eat" is a frequently heard complaint.

Normally, appetite begins to decrease during the latter part of the first year of life. It decreases to its lowest level between 18 and 36 months and does not increase significantly until 5 or 6 years of age.

Between the ages of 18 and 36 months the child is also going through a state called psychologic negativism (see Chapter 21), during which everything, including eating, is received with a "no." During this period the child's growth rate decreases, as does his weight gain, so that the child loses his "baby fat." The child also becomes extremely interested in the world, which offers expanded fields of exploration, and he does not like to waste time eating.

Diagnostically, the child needs evaluation only if he is disproportionate from his peers—for example, a child at the ninetieth percentile for height but at the third percentile in weight. If there is a marked change in the child's own growth curve or if there are other signs or symptoms, such as delayed development, an abdominal mass, or a significant heart murmur, evaluation is also needed.

During this period when the appetite is normally poor, parents need education as to what is occurring and reassurance that everything is normal. Furthermore, the pediatric nurse practitioner should stress the fact that it is healthier to be somewhat underweight than overweight and that overweight infants and children seem to have a greater tendency toward obesity as adults. If the pediatric nurse practitioner alerts the parents to the decrease in appetite, parents will have little concern when it occurs; it is far easier to counsel them before the fact than to reassure them afterward.

NUTRITIONAL COUNSELING

Since dietitians and nutritionists have specialized training in nutrition, they are better able than the nurse practitioner to counsel patients who should follow special diets. However, for the majority of patients the pediatric nurse practitioner should be able to counsel mothers regarding the diets of their children by following certain general guidelines.

Food can be divided into four groups: (1) milk group, (2) meat group, (3) vegetable and fruit group, and (4) bread and cereal group.

The milk group includes milk, ice cream, cheese, and other dairy products. The meat group includes meats, fish, poultry, eggs, beans, and nuts. The vegetable and fruit group includes dark green or yellow vegetables and citrus fruits or tomatoes. The bread and cereal group contains bread, crackers, potatoes, and rice.

A child's daily diet should include approximately four servings from the vegetable and fruit groups and four from the bread and cereal group. It should also contain two servings from the meat group and two to four glasses of milk each day (or a substitute from the same group) not to exceed 32 ounces per day.

INFANT FEEDING

In feedings, as in other matters concerning a child, the mother should be encouraged to make her own decisions whenever possible. The advantages and disadvantages of breast feeding and formula feeding, and the differences among formulas should be discussed with the mother. She should make the final decision as to what type of feeding she will use. The pediatric nurse practitioner should make the mother aware, however, that certain faulty techniques, such as propping of the bottle, could result in aspiration and certainly will deprive the infant of the emotional gratification associated with feeding. Allowing the mother to make her own decisions demands that the nurse practitioner invest both time and energy in counseling; the feeling of competence gained by the mother and the rapport established will be well worth the investment. Dictatorial methods that leave no room for the mother's choice of alternatives foster a feeling of dependency in the mother.

Whether infants receive breast milk or artificial feedings, it is best to have them on a modified demand feeding (flexible regular) schedule. In general, babies empty their stomach in about 3 hours and those on breast milk empty their stomach somewhat faster than those on artificial formulas. Thus, infants are usually fed every 3 to 4 hours, especially during the first 2 or 3 months of life.

Although opinions are numerous and the rigidity of some schedules concerning the addition of solid food to the diet is surprising, it is important to realize that infants obtain adequate nutrition from breast milk or from their formula, except for vitamins, for the first 4 months of life.

Often, in our culture, mothers will be anxious to start solids early. There is no harm in introducing cereals or strained foods as early as 3 to 4 weeks of age; however, the mother should be warned that the baby's swallowing mechanism is geared to sucking and that he may tend to spit the food out. The mother also needs to be told that whether or not the infant takes a few spoonfuls of "solids" at this young age will not make any difference in his state of health and that food allergies may develop more frequently with early introduction of numerous foods.

Food allergies develop more often during the first year of life than at any other time. Therefore, only one new food is introduced at one time and the mother is advised to wait at least 1 week before introducing another new food. When symptoms of allergy develop (diarrhea, vomiting, or skin rash), the last food to be introduced is discontinued first and is frequently found to be the offending agent. Highly allergenic foods should be avoided during the first year. Foods to be avoided include corn, citrus fruits and juices, tomatoes, egg white, fish, chocolate, and nuts. In families where allergies are common, wheat products are also best avoided and in some cases allergists may recommend the avoidance of all food except for breast milk or formula for the first 3 or 4 months of life.

Soft solid foods should be started by 3 to 4 months of age or when the consumption of formula reaches 32 ounces a day. Cereal with milk or formula is usually the first solid food fed, followed by pureed vegetables, fruits, meat, and egg yolk. Although egg yolk is a good source of iron, its usefulness has been questioned because of its high cholesterol content and its possible relation with arteriosclerosis.

There is no best sequence for the introduction of solids but meat or egg yolk should be introduced by 3 to 4 months or earlier if the infant reaches a milk consumption of 32 ounces per day. It is important to provide a good intake of a food rich in iron by 5 to 6 months of age, so that iron is available for hemoglobin synthesis. By 6 months of age the maternal iron supply is no longer adequate.

By the end of the first year infants should be allowed to feed themselves with food which they can handle with their fingers, such as french fries, hot dogs, cut vegetables, and crackers.

Breast feeding. Breast feeding is the preferred way, physically and psychologically, to feed infants for the first few months of life, even though breast-fed babies may gain weight more slowly during the first few weeks of life. The nurse practitioner also should know that bottle feeding with properly prepared formula given with love and care is almost as satisfactory as breast feeding. It may be preferable in some cases when mothers do not want to breast feed their offspring.

To prevent breast feeding failures, it should be remembered that the most satisfactory stimulus for milk production is the emptying of the breast. Therefore, if a mother gives the infant many supplementary bottles, her milk supply is going to diminish. Also the lactating mother needs an adequate fluid intake, particularly after 4 to 6 weeks when the infant is emptying both breasts at a feeding.

Artificial formulas. Cow's milk is higher in protein and lower in carbohydrates than human milk but both have 20 calories per ounce. Therefore, in order to make cow's milk similar to human milk, most artificial formulas are based on diluting cow's milk with water and adding carbohydrates.

The caloric requirement of an infant is approximately 50 to 55 calories per pound per day or 110 calories per kilogram of body weight. One way to prepare a quart (32 ounces) of artificial formula is to mix 13 ounces (one can) of evaporated milk with 17 ounces of water and 2 tablespoons of carbohydrates, such as commercially available syrup.

Most commercially prepared formulas are based on cow's milk with added vitamins. Children who are allergic to cow's milk require some other form of feeding. The two most common milk substitutes are soybean preparations or mixtures of amino acids with fats, carbohydrates, and vitamins. These are prepared to provide 20 calories per ounce. Meat-based formulas are also available for infants who cannot tolerate milk.

PATHOLOGIC NUTRITIONAL STATES

In the United States today there are two clinically important nutritional diseases in the pediatric age group: iron deficiency anemia of infancy and obesity.

Iron deficiency anemia of infancy. Iron deficiency anemia of infancy is the most common anemia in pediatrics in the United States today. It occurs most commonly between the ages of 9 and 18 months, not only because maternal iron stores last only for 6 months (less in premature babies), but also because infants are growing very fast during that period of their lives. Many infants obtain most of their calories from iron-poor food such as milk and not from iron-rich food such as meat or egg yolk.

Children with a severe iron deficiency anemia tend to be chubby, pale, and irritable and usually give a history of excessive milk intake and poor intake of solids.

In iron deficiency anemia the hemoglobin is below 10 grams per 100 ml; the red blood cells are hypochromic and microcytic (low in hemoglobin and small), and serum iron is reduced.

Iron deficiency anemia is usually treated by the oral administration of iron salts such as ferrous sulfate and by counseling regarding proper nutrition.

Iron deficiency anemia is a totally preventable condition; all premature infants, twins, and chronically ill infants should receive supplemental iron, usually 1 mg per kilogram of body weight of ferrous sulfate or its equivalent daily. When the child is already anemic due to iron deficiency, the dose of ferrous sulfate should be increased to 6 mg per kilogram of body weight per day. Several commercial formulas are now supplemented to provide 12 mg of iron per quart as prophylaxis for such infants.

For infants born with adequate iron stores—healthy full-term newborns— the introduction of food containing iron, such as meat and egg yolk, at 4 or 5 months of age suffices to prevent iron deficiency anemia. Milk is a very poor source of iron and no child should drink more than 24 to 32 ounces a day. If the child is already anemic, he should be given 24 ounces a day, so that he will be hungry and eat foods rich in iron.

Obesity. Obesity is a condition in which there is an increase in body fat. Since methods to determine body fat are cumbersome, body weight is the commonly accepted criterion to determine obesity.

Obesity is usually related to excessive food intake, reduced activity, or both. Obesity caused by endocrine disorders is extremely rare and it is usually associated with other endocrinologic signs, such as high blood pressure, striae, and buffalo humps. Thyroid disease is often blamed for obesity and many overweight adolescents receive medicinal thyroid unnecessarily.

Diagnosis of obesity is made either by inspection or by plotting the patient's height and weight in a standard chart. An accurate history of food intake is very difficult to obtain because obese patients make extensive use of denial in areas related to obesity.

In the treatment of obesity the purpose is to reverse the positive energy balance, or excessive food intake with decreased activity. Unfortunately, none of the methods used to cure obesity has been even moderately successful.

Some of the approaches used are (1) drugs to decrease appetite, which seem to be useful for only 2 or 3 weeks; (2) clubs or groups such as Weight Watchers, which provide group reinforcement and which seem to be somewhat beneficial; (3) fasting, which is one of the newest approaches (however, the long-term results are not yet available); and (4) psychiatric help individually or in groups, a technique that is also of limited value.

Obesity is life threatening since it increases the incidence of arteriosclerosis, high blood pressure, diabetes, and other potentially lethal diseases. It has a poor prognosis and in its management the health worker usually plays only a supportive role. The pediatric practitioners are in a unique position to attempt to arrest the problem early, since there is more and more evidence indicating that obese young children become fat older children who in turn become fat adults.

Chapter 10

HEALTH SUPERVISION

Health supervision is an essential part of pediatrics, which, more than any other clinical specialty, has been concerned with preventive health practices.

In health supervision the goals are promotion of general health through counseling; prevention of illness through the use of immunizations; early diagnosis of asymptomatic illnesses to permit early treatment and prevent complications; early diagnosis and treatment of symptomatic illnesses to prevent complications; and prevention of unnecessary disability from known chronic illness.

The techniques used in health supervision are:

1. History and physical examination
2. Developmental assessment
3. Screening tests (clinical and laboratory)
4. Immunization
5. Counseling

The history and physical examination are useful in detecting both symptomatic and asymptomatic illnesses. They also offer an excellent opportunity to relate to the child and his family in order to detect incipient or more advanced psychologic problems. It is well to remember that not every child brought to a health facility needs a complete history and physical examination. It does make a difference whether the child is brought for a yearly health supervision visit, at which time he needs a complete evaluation, or if he is brought to determine the outcome of an acute illness (see Chapters 2 and 3).

Evaluation of growth rate is an important part of the physical examination of children, since chronically ill children do not grow well (see Chapter 5).

Developmental assessment through the use of the history of developmental milestones or a structured test, such as the Denver Developmental Scale, is important in evaluating neuromuscular development, a significant indicator of the development of the brain (see Chapter 6).

There are several screening tests that are part of the health appraisal

Table 4. Health supervision schedule used at Cardinal Glennon Memorial Hospital for Children

First 24 hours	History and newborn examination, Guthrie test or urine PKU after 2 to 3 days of age
2 months	History and physical examination, DPT and OPV, urine PKU
3 months	DPT
4 months	History and physical examination, DPT, and OPV
6 months	History and physical examination, OPV, urinalysis
12 months	History and physical examination, tuberculin test (read Tuberculin and give live measles vaccine), hemoglobin and sickle cell preparation
15-18 months	History and physical examination, DPT, OPV, and smallpox
2-2½ years	Rubella vaccine, urine (coproporphyrin)
3 years	History and physical examination, tuberculin test
4-6 years	History and physical examination with developmental assessment (DDS), DPT, OPV, smallpox and TBC tests, vision and hearing screening tests, urinalysis (girls; yearly)
7-11 years	History and physical examination yearly
12-15 years	History and physical examination yearly, dT, smallpox, mumps, and tuberculin test

Notes: A. Do not immunize children who are febrile or acutely ill as with a "cold." B. Oral polio (OPV) for children older than 1 year old with no previous polio vaccine. Give 2 doses 2 months apart and a third dose 1 year later. C. After 15 years of age dT should be given every 10 years and smallpox every 3-10 years. D. Tuberculin should be administered yearly and not together with live virus vaccines.

of children. Some are clinical tests such as the vision and hearing tests (see Chapter 4); others are laboratory tests such as urinalysis, the ferric chloride or Guthrie tests for phenylketonuria, or tests to determine hemoglobin values (see Chapter 7).

Immunization materials are the best tools known to prevent illnesses. Available immunization material, as well as the indication and contraindications for their administration, is discussed in Chapter 8.

An integral part of health supervision must always be developmental and emotional counseling (see Chapters 5, 6, and 9).

Although schedules followed in health supervision in different clinics or physicians' offices are based on the same general goals, they are not and should not be exactly the same in every facility. The schedules should be geared to specific characteristics and needs of each community depending on the prevalence of different illnesses and the available facilities.

Table 4 shows the schedule for health supervision used at Cardinal Glennon Memorial Hospital for Children (St. Louis).

Chapter 11
EMERGENCIES

Pediatric nurse practitioners should always be able to recognize and evaluate the severity of emergencies so that they may institute immediate, and at times lifesaving, therapy and obtain appropriate help.

The nurse practitioner should become familiar with cardiorespiratory failure, dehydration, diabetic emergencies, convulsions, meningitis, accidents (injuries, poisoning, burns), and animal bites.

CARDIORESPIRATORY FAILURE

A patient with no heartbeat may have either true cardiac arrest (ventricular standstill) or ventricular fibrillation. Ventricular standstill is often the end result of complete anoxia, which in children is most frequently caused by severe croup, aspiration of a foreign body, or drowning. Ventricular fibrillation is most frequently the result of electric shock.

Most croups are viral and do not produce complete respiratory obstruction. However, a few are caused by *Hemophilus influenzae;* clinically these show epiglottitis and often lead to complete respiratory obstruction. Aspiration of foreign bodies may also cause complete obstruction of the airway if the foreign body is lodged in the larynx or trachea. Drowning leads to respiratory obstruction through reflex spasm of the vocal cords.

The *first* thing that must be done in cases of cardiorespiratory arrest is to establish an airway. This is done by suctioning of upper airway secretions and ventilating through (1) mouth-to-mouth breathing, (2) positive pressure breathing with a tight mask, or (3) intratracheal intubation with positive pressure breathing into the intratracheal tube with short bursts of air. Connection of the intratracheal tube to a bag (such as the Ambu bag) facilitates positive pressure breathing. If intubation is impossible a tracheotomy needs to be performed. In an emergency a high tracheotomy or crycothyroidectomy is easier. In a crycothyroidectomy an opening is made surgically into the upper airway below the Adam's apple.

Secondly, since the absence of a heartbeat could be the result of ventricular fibrillation or ventricular arrest, give a sharp blow on the chest over the sternum. If the patient has ventricular fibrillation this maneuver may convert him back to a normal rhythm. Since, on the other hand, absence of heartbeat

59

could be the result of ventricular arrest, cardiac massage needs to be initiated by straight downward pressure of the body of the sternum. Cardiac massage in infants is performed by applying jerky pressure with the distal part of the thumb on the xyphoid. In older children and adults it should be done with the heel of the hand, one hand supporting and aiding the other until femoral pulses are obtained. For cardiac massage the patient needs to be on a hard surface such as a board or the floor. As soon as possible an electrocardiogram should be obtained and if it shows that the patient is fibrillating, an electrical defibrillator should be used.

Certain drugs, such as sodium bicarbonate, epinephrine, and calcium gluconate, are utilized in cardiorespiratory arrest to counteract the cardiac inactivity as well as the metabolic changes, such as acidosis (decreased pH) and hyperkalemia (increased potassium level), which occur. Sodium bicarbonate counteracts the acidosis, calcium gluconate the hyperkalemia, and epinephrine is a myocardial stimulant. Sodium bicarbonate may be administered as a 0.89 milliequivalent per ml solution in a dose of 5 to 20 ml depending on the size of the patient; calcium gluconate may be used in a 10 percent solution, 1 to 5 ml, depending on the size of the patient. Epinephrine is used in a concentration of 1:10,000 (the 1:1,000 commercially available solution diluted 1 to 10 with normal saline) in a dose of 1 to 5 ml depending on the size of the patient. All of these drugs should be administered intravenously or intracardially.

DEHYDRATION

Dehydration is often the result of diarrhea and vomiting and is usually not as acute an emergency as cardiorespiratory failure.

Clinically, dehydration is classified into *mild,* 5 percent, or the earliest clinically detectable dehydration; *moderate,* 8 percent, in which definite signs of dehydration such as decreased skin turgor, dry mucosa, sunken fontanels, and decreased eye pressure are present; and *severe,* or the greatest dehydration compatible with life in which all of the above described signs of dehydration are present and the child is in shock. In all dehydration urine volume is decreased and thus the frequency and volume of urination is an important point to evaluate in the history.

Pediatric nurse practitioners should be able to recognize mild dehydration in order to prevent further dehydration. Mildly dehydrated children should not receive solid foods or milk. They should be given a dilute electrolyte solution, such as root beer, ginger ale, gelatin water, or half-strength orange juice. Some authorities prefer to give the patient small sips of coke syrup or the syrup of canned pears or peaches before dilute electrolyte solutions are given. Very concentrated electrolyte solutions, such as full-strength skimmed milk, or home-made electrolyte solutions, such as a mixture of water, sugar, and salt, should be avoided because the patient may be overloaded with salt. This

Table 5. Normal serum electrolyte values

Sodium	136-143	milliequivalents per liter
Potassium	4.1-5.6	milliequivalents per liter
Chloride	98-106	milliequivalents per liter
Bicarbonate	23-30	milliequivalents per liter
pH	7.3-7.45	

may lead to a more severe type of dehydration—hypertonic dehydration—which often produces brain damage.

After the child is tolerating the dilute electrolyte solution well, he should be given a bland diet consisting of gelatin, rice cereal, bananas, applesauce, saltine crackers, chicken, and turkey.

Moderate and severe dehydration require intravenous therapy. In an emergency, intravenous therapy should be started immediately with an electrolyte solution. Such electrolyte solution will expand the extracellular volume. Examples of suitable electrolyte solutions for intravenous therapy include normal saline, 5 percent dextrose in one-fourth to full-strength saline, and Ringer's lactate. A safe dose of normal saline with which to begin intravenous therapy in a child with severe dehydration is 30 ml per kilogram of body weight administered as fast as it will run into the vein. Initial intravenous solution should not contain potassium. Potassium should be added after the child urinates.

The pediatric nurse practitioner does not need to know specific details of fluid and electrolyte therapy but should become familiar with the normal serum electrolyte values (see Table 5) and some basic principles utilized in calculating fluid and electrolyte therapy.

In fluid and electrolyte treatment the amount of fluid required is equal to the sum of the amount required for body maintenance plus amounts required to replenish previous deficit and current losses.

Maintenance fluids consist of the amount of fluid and electrolyte necessary to maintain normal obligatory body losses. Since infants are born with water excess, and since water requirements depend on the metabolic rate (see Chapter 5), the amount of water required for maintenance is approximately 60 ml per kilogram of body weight per day in the first week of life. This amount increases to a peak at 80 to 100 ml per kilogram of body per day weight between the ages of 1 week and 1 year and then constantly decreases to about 40 ml per kilogram of body weight during adolescence. The amount of sodium and potassium are approximately 1 to 2 milliequivalent per kilogram of body weight per day. Deficit and current losses vary considerably depending on the situation, and each clinical situation needs individual consideration.

CONVULSIONS

Convulsions are common in children and account for numerous emergency room visits. The causes of convulsions are numerous (Chapter 20). Regardless of the etiology of convulsions the first step is to establish an airway if it is obstructed with secretions or if the tongue is in the way; aspiration must be avoided by positioning the patient on his side. The nurse practitioner must also prevent the patient from hurting himself, but must be careful in attempting to restrain the patient too strenuously because he could be injured in the process. Drugs such as phenobarbital, diazepam, and paraldehyde are essential in the management of convulsions.

MENINGITIS

Headache, fever, and sometimes convulsions are presenting complaints in meningitis. However, the young child with meningitis is more often seen with fever and paradoxical irritability (he wants to be left alone because when he is held his spinal nerve roots are stretched and become painful).

The physical examination classically reveals stiff neck and Kernig's and Brudzinski's signs, all of which are signs of meningeal irritation (see Chapter 20). The younger the patient the less likely he is to present the classical signs of meningitis, but the greater his chance of having a tense, bulging fontanel.

If meningitis is suspected, a lumbar puncture should be performed and the fluid examined as described in Chapter 7. Meningitis classically is manifested by increased polymorphonuclear leukocytes and decreased sugar content of the fluid. If evidence of bacterial meningitis is found on the examination of the cerebrospinal fluid, appropriate antibiotic therapy needs to be instituted. Currently, the most widely used antibiotic in meningitis before final bacteriologic diagnosis is made by culture is ampicillin given intravenously. However, in newborns the disease is often caused by coliform bacilli, which are not sensitive to ampicillin, and other antibiotics are usually utilized.

ACCIDENTS

Accidents are the leading cause of death between the ages of 1 and 24 years. Accidents are second only to infection as the cause of acute morbidity and visits to physicians' offices during childhood.

Some of the most frequently occurring accidents are motor vehicle accidents, falls, burns, drowning, and poisoning.

Accidental injuries. Serious accidental injuries are most commonly caused by motor vehicles and falls. In dealing with serious accidental injuries the nurse practitioner must first make sure that the airway is open and that the heart is beating. If there is cardiorespiratory failure proceed as previously described in this chapter.

Secondly, bleeding must be controlled, which is generally done through direct pressure on the bleeding site. The child must then be examined for evidence of internal injury, such as ruptured liver, spleen, kidney, or intracranial injury (see Chapter 3). Subsequently the child needs to be evaluated for fractures. If fractures are suspected, the area should be immobilized by whatever means of splinting are available. This is of utmost importance in neck and spine injuries where spinal cord injury can be prevented if proper immobilization is instituted.

Poisoning. There are about 4,000 accidental poisoning fatalities in the United States each year, and half of these occur in children. The most common age for accidental poisoning in children is between 1 and 4 years of age. The ingested substances can be divided into medicinal and nonmedicinal substances. The medicinal substances include aspirin, iron-containing products (such as vitamins with iron), and tranquilizers. The nonmedicinal products include household products such as furniture polish, cleansing and laundry products, and drain cleaners, as well as cosmetics and insecticides.

Education is of extreme importance to prevent ingestion of both medicinal and nonmedicinal products. Parents need basic information regarding the dangers of their children ingesting common drugs, such as aspirin, iron tablets, and tranquilizers. They should be advised to keep especially large quantities of medications in a locked cabinet and should be taught how to prevent nonmedicinal ingestion. For example, products such as drain cleaners and dishwasher detergent should not be stored under the sink and they should never be put in soft drink bottles. Parents and others caring for children also need awareness that ingestions most frequently occur during mid-morning and most often during times of family crisis when the child feels deserted, such as during hospitalization of another member of the family or after a death in the family.

When poisoning has already occurred the treatment consists of elimination of the poisonous substance, administration of specific antidotes, and support of vital functions such as respirations, heart, blood pressure, and temperature. The nearest poison control center should be consulted immediately if there are any questions regarding the effect of the ingested substance or the management of the patient.

Elimination of the poison is accomplished by either gastric lavage or by inducing vomiting with an emetic. Ten to 15 ml of Ipecac syrup orally is the most frequently used emetic. This dose is repeated in 20 to 30 minutes if no vomiting occurs. If vomiting still does not occur, gastric lavage should be performed, not only because of the ingested poison itself, but also because Ipecac is cardiotoxic and therefore should be eliminated. Activated charcoal increases elimination of the toxic product in both lavage and vomiting; however, the charcoal may also absorb the Ipecac and render it ineffective as an emetic.

Do not induce vomiting or perform gastric lavage if the patient has ingested caustic agents or petroleum distillates. Some examples of caustic agents are toilet bowl cleaners, drain cleaners, laundry soap, ammonia, rust removers, laundry bleaches, and dishwasher detergent. Some petroleum distillates are furniture polish, kerosene, oil, gasoline, and paint thinners. Lavage or vomiting after ingestion of caustic agents may cause perforation of the esophagus. Pneumonia, which is usually acquired through aspiration, is the most worrisome problem of petroleum distillate ingestion and is commonly induced during vomiting or gastric lavage. Therefore, these two procedures should not be done, especially if the amount of petroleum distillate ingested is small.

Induction of vomiting should also be avoided when the patient is comatose or has ingested a substance that may induce convulsions, since emesis may precipitate convulsions. One must also be careful in performing gastric lavage in a comatose patient because of the danger of aspiration. In such cases it is often necessary to use an intratracheal tube with a cuff. If gastric lavage is necessary in a patient who is convulsing, convulsions need to be well controlled first.

Administration of specific antidotes against the ingested poison, if indicated, is important; however, unfortunately, most poisons do not have specific antidotes. Poison control information centers should be consulted for specific information regarding an ingested substance of questionable toxicity.

Supportive measures are of utmost importance in poisoning. For example, if the toxic product produces depression of respiration, respiration needs to be assisted; if the toxic product produces hypotension, the blood pressure needs to be maintained.

Lead poisoning. Lead poisoning, because it differs epidemiologically from other cases of poisoning, deserves individual consideration. Lead poisoning in children is most often caused by ingestion of lead base paint or putty. It occurs most often in children 1 to 5 years of age who live in houses that were built before World War II and have not been well maintained so that there is crumbling paint and plaster. Occasionally, toys or cribs are repainted with lead paint. Little children frequently chew on loose paint chips, window sills, or plaster. Lead gradually accumulates in the body and affects the function of many organs especially the kidneys, brain, and bone marrow. The nurse practitioner should routinely inquire about the chewing or eating of paint or plaster when examining children in this age group, especially if they live in old, run-down houses. Early symptoms are often overlooked because they are vague and nonspecific. Symptoms include anorexia, listlessness, constipation, difficulty in coordination, ataxia, or loss of recently acquired skills. These symptoms should alert the practitioner to the possibility of lead poisoning and appropriate laboratory studies should be obtained.

Blood lead levels, hematocrit values, urinalysis, urine coproporphyrin determinations, and radiographs of long bones are indicated. Growth arrest lines shown in radiographs of long bones are sometimes referred to as "lead lines," but they are really due to temporary cessation of growth. A blood level above 0.040 mg per 100 ml indicates increased exposure to lead. Elevated

Table 6. Guide for postexposure antirabies prophylaxis*

Biting animal	Status at time of attack	Treatment exposure		
		No lesion	Mild†	Severe†
Dog or cat	Healthy	None	None‡	S‡
	Signs suggestive of rabies	None	V§	S+V§
	Escaped or unknown	None	V	S+V
	Rabid	None	S+V	S+V
Skunk, fox, raccoon, coyote, bat	Regard as rabid in un- provoked attack	None	S+V	S+V

*Recommendations of the Public Health Service Advisory Committee on Immunization Practices and the American Academy of Pediatrics, Committee on Infectious Diseases published in the *Morbidity and Mortality Weekly Report*, Vol. 16, No. 19 week ending May 13, 1967 and in the Report of the Committee on Infectious Diseases, American Academy of Pediatrics, 1970. These recommendations are intended only as a guide. They may be modified according to knowledge of the species of biting animal and circumstances surrounding the biting incident.

†"Severe"—multiple or deep puncture wounds and any bites on head, face, neck, hands or fingers. "Mild" —scratches, lacerations, wounds, contamination with salvia and single bites on the body in areas other than "severe."

‡Begin vaccine at first sign of rabies in biting dog or cat during holding period (perferably 7 to 10 days).

§Discontinue vaccine if biting dog or cat is healthy 5 days after exposure or if acceptable laboratory negativity has been demonstrated in animal killed at time of attack. If observed animal dies after 5 days and brain is positive for rabies, resume treatment.

V = Rabies vaccine.

S = Antirabies serum.

blood levels should prompt referral to the municipal housing authority in order to investigate the source of exposure to lead and facilitate its removal. If a child has symptoms, or if the blood lead level is greater than 50 μg per 100 ml, the physician should decide what further studies or treatment are indicated. Signs and symptoms of severe chronic lead poisoning are abdominal pain or those signs and symptoms associated with increased intracranial pressure, such as vomiting, convulsions, and coma.

Burns. Burns are among the most common accidents in children. In case of a burn, the area should be immediately cooled by placing the area under cold running water when possible or by application of cool wet cloths.

Burns are usually divided into three degrees: first degree, in which there is redness of the skin; second degree, when there is formation of blisters; and third degree, when the area is insensitive to pain because the nerve endings are burned. Currently, first and second degree burns are called partial-thickness burns, and the third degree burns are full-thickness burns.

Burns are a problem because of dehydration, infection, and residual scarring. After the initial treatment described above, expert medical and surgical help is necessary.

Animal bites. Animal bites can be divided into insect bites or stings and larger animal bites. Each of them has specific problems.

Although insect bites usually produce no more problem than a small area of redness and swelling around the site of the sting, a few persons who are extremely sensitive develop rapid, life-threatening swelling of the airway tissues (laryngeal mucosa). In these cases the administration of 0.1 to 0.3 ml of epinephrine (1:1,000) subcutaneously may be necessary. If, after an insect bite such as a bee, wasp, or hornet sting, the patient develops signs of systemic or generalized allergy such as urticaria, wheezing, or swelling of an entire extremity, he should be referred to an allergist for hyposensitization injections in order to prevent a possible fatal outcome of subsequent reactions to insect sting.

Wound infection, tetanus, and rabies are possible complications of larger animal bites. Extensive washing with soap and water soon after the bite is always important since it decreases the possibility of infection, tetanus, and rabies by removal of the offending organisms.

An accurate history with subsequent administration of appropriate tetanus immunization or tetanus hyperimmune serum is necessary in order to prevent tetanus. Rabies immunization is administered according to the rules stated in Table 6, which are the recommendations of the American Academy of Pediatrics and the American Public Health Association.

Chapter 12
THE RESPIRATORY SYSTEM

In man, and particularly in children, bacterial and viral respiratory infections are the greatest single cause of morbidity or illness. The present chapter will first discuss two common presenting symptoms of respiratory problems, cough and epistaxis, and will then consider some of the respiratory illnesses that the pediatrician most often encounters, such as pharyngitis, otitis media, laryngotracheobronchitis, bronchiolitis, asthma, and pneumonia.

COUGH

Cough, a frequent symptom of acute or chronic respiratory tract irritation, may be produced by a multiplicity of causes. Environmental dryness, material in the respiratory tract such as secretions or foreign bodies, bronchospasms, or psychogenic problems may all result in coughing.

Environmental dryness irritates the respiratory mucosa and thus causes coughing. Dryness becomes a considerable problem especially in the winter when houses are heated without proper humidification. Ideal humidity is around 50 percent.

Although dryness by itself accounts for a great deal of coughing, other causes should be considered. In children with cough the presence of a foreign body is always a likely possibility. Increased secretions caused by respiratory infections with or without bronchospasm may also produce coughing. In these cases coughing, aided by proper humidity, has a protective value, since it clears the respiratory tract of abnormal secretions. The value of expectorants, except for bronchodilators in the case of asthmatic bronchospasms, is questionable. Coughing may also be a somatic expression of anxiety or other nervous tensions.

EPISTAXIS

The site of epistaxis, or nosebleed, in children is almost always found in the mucosa over the anterior portion of the septum. Epistaxis is often caused by minor trauma such as picking the nose. It is also common in the winter when the nasal mucosa is exposed to low humidity due to heating without proper humidification. Epistaxis rarely warrants further diagnostic investigation, unless it is recurrent or difficult to stop.

Most epistaxes respond to pressure-pinching of the nose; at times vaso-constrictor medications need to be used, and on very infrequent occasions packing of the nose is necessary.

PHARYNGITIS

Physical examination and awareness of particular viruses and bacteria that produce illnesses in a community at a particular time should help in the diagnosis of pharyngitis.

The practitioner must first determine whether the pharyngitis is bacterial, in which the major pathogen is group A beta hemolytic *Streptococcus,* or viral. Although bacterial infections cannot always be differentiated from viral infections by visual inspection, an intensely red pharynx with exudate suggests the infection is bacterial. Similarly, small ulcers on the pillars of the pharynx and soft palate are almost always viral in origin. The patient with viral pharyngitis usually has few other complaints, his temperature is normal or only slightly elevated, and there is only slight tenderness and enlargement of the cervical lymph nodes. Bacterial pharyngitis is most often associated with generalized malaise, fever, and enlarged tender lymph nodes. Infectious mononucleosis may also produce pharyngitis with exudate and should be considered if the lymph nodes are especially prominent or if the fever and malaise are out of proportion to the appearance of the throat.

The traditional method of determining the origin of an infection based on the white blood cell count (decreased in viral illnesses and elevated in bacterial infections) is unfortunately not very helpful in differentiating viral from bacterial pharyngitis. In infectious mononucleosis the white blood cell count is either normal or elevated, but the differential white blood cell count shows "atypical" immature lymphocytes (see Chapter 13). Cultures are definitive in making an etiologic diagnosis. Cultures may be sent to a laboratory or may be done as an office or clinic procedure (see Chapter 7).

The treatment of choice for acute streptococcal pharyngitis is administration of penicillin for 10 days. When patients are allergic to penicillin other antibiotics such as erythromycin should be used. In viral acute pharyngitis, the treatment is only symptomatic—aspirin to control fever and soothing throat lozenges.

OTITIS MEDIA

Acute otitis media is usually caused by *Pneumococcus* or group A beta hemolytic *Streptococcus* in children 4 years of age or older. *Pneumococcus* or *Hemophilus influenzae* causes the disease in children 6 months to 4 years of age. Otitis media may also be caused by viruses. The diagnosis of otitis media is made by inspection of the tympanic membrane, which becomes red or "beefy" with distorted landmarks (see Chapter 3). If the canal is impacted with wax that occludes the tympanic membrane, the wax should be removed (see Chapter 3). Although crying may cause the eardrums to become red, the landmarks of the tympanic membrane remain normal if the child does not have otitis media.

Since bacterial otitis media cannot be differentiated from viral otitis media except through culture of the middle ear, antibiotics to cover the most likely bacterial organism in different age groups are usually prescribed. Among the antibiotics most commonly utilized are ampicillin for children 6 months to 4 years and penicillin for children older than 4 years. According to some investigators, oral decongestants can be of help in the management of acute otitis media by encouraging drainage through the eustachian tube.

A return visit to determine whether or not there is residual serous otitis caused by the presence of fluid in the middle ear is of utmost importance. If drainage of the eustachian tube is poor, chronic serous otitis media can occur as a sequela of acute otitis media. Chronic serous otitis media is a treatable cause of hearing loss in children. A normal hearing test after an episode of otitis is of extreme significance in determining whether or not the otitis has been completely resolved (see Chapter 4).

In the presence of chronic serous otitis media or when there is transient serous otitis media after an acute infection, the tympanic membrane is red and the normal landmarks, such as the umbo and light reflex, become distorted. At times air bubbles are observed behind the tympanic membrane.

In the treatment of chronic serous otitis media, a high environmental humidity vaporizer or humidifier should be used. Maneuvers to inflate the eustachian tube (such as swallowing with the nose pinched) should be performed, and oral decongestants such as vasoconstrictor antihistamine combinations should also be used. Should there be no response to the above conservative methods, the patient may need a complete allergic evaluation to determine possible allergic etiology. In some cases surgical procedures such as adenoidectomy or tympanotomy with insertion of prosthetic tubes may be needed in order to artificially ventilate the middle ear.

LARYNGOTRACHEOBRONCHITIS (CROUP)

Croup is an inflammation of the larynx. Most croups are caused by viral infection and a few by bacterial infection.

Viral croup is usually slower in progression and the patient appears less ill than the patient with bacterial croup. In bacterial croup the child looks very sick and the onset of the illness is quite sudden. Marked respiratory difficulty within 12 hours from the onset of symptoms and a cherry-like, red epiglottis are characteristic signs of bacterial croup (see Chapter 3). A child with inspiratory stridor needs to be examined sitting up, since the chances of producing complete obstruction due to a vocal cord spasm in patients with epiglottitis are greater if the child is lying down.

Bacterial croup is much more dangerous than viral croup because a high percentage result in complete obstruction and require a tracheotomy; viral croup almost never causes complete obstruction.

Both viral and bacterial croups are associated with "croupy cough," a high pitched cough, which reminds the examiner of the barking of a dog. Inspiratory stridor, a high pitched noise, is heard on inspiration. In severe cases retraction of the suprasternal notch and intercostal spaces occurs on inspiration.

Both viral and bacterial croup need to be treated with high humidity through the use of a humidifier, vaporizer, or croup tent (croupette). If such equipment is not available, taking the child into the bathroom with the hot water shower open provides significant humidity. Bacterial croup also requires antibiotics. The most frequently used today is ampicillin because it is effective against *Hemophilus influenzae*. However, in spite of humidity and antibiotics, patients with bacterial croup must be carefully watched so that a tracheotomy can be done immediately if complete obstruction occurs.

BRONCHIOLITIS AND ASTHMA

Bronchiolitis is an inflammatory expiratory obstruction of acute onset occurring in the first 2 years of life. The child behaves as does an older child with asthma. Therefore, on physical examination he has a prolonged obstructed expiration with trapped air producing a hyperresonant percussion note. Expiratory wheezes are heard upon auscultation of the chest.

Bronchiolitis is usually caused by an acute viral infection with respiratory syncytial virus, although it may be caused by *Hemophilus influenzae.*

Children with viral bronchiolitis need humidity and supportive care. If the bronchiolitis is produced by bacteria an antibiotic such as ampicillin which will cover *Hemophilus influenzae* is needed in addition.

Asthma is a respiratory obstruction produced by bronchospasm and hypersecretion of the lower respiratory tract. The signs on physical examination are similar to those of severe bronchiolitis—expiratory obstruction, trapped air, a hyperresonant percussion note, and expiratory wheezes upon auscultation.

Asthma has an allergic basis; however, a number of factors in a child's life may trigger acute attacks. Thus, emotions, infections, or exposure to a large antigenic dose such as breathing air with a high content of allergens (for example, ragweed) may precipitate an acute asthmatic episode.

In children between the ages of 2 and 8 years, an acute infection of the respiratory tract frequently precipitates an attack. In older children and adults asthma is very frequently seasonal, improves with hyposensitization, and is usually associated with specific environmental allergens such as ragweed.

The treatment of asthma consists of humidity and hydration; administration of bronchodilators such as epinephrine and aminophylline; antibiotics, should there be a bacterial infection; and, in extreme cases, corticosteroids. In very extreme cases sedation, paralysis (with morphine and curare), and artificial ventilation with the aid of mechanical devices may be necessary. Children with frequent episodes of asthma should be evaluated by an allergist.

PNEUMONIA

Pneumonia is an acute inflammation of the lung and is caused by an infectious agent. Although often caused by *Pneumococcus,* other organisms such as *Mycoplasma, Staphylococcus aureus, Mycobacterium tuberculosum, Histoplasma,* and viruses may also produce pneumonia.

The child with pneumonia gives a variable history. In older children there is fever, cough, chest pain, and sputum production. In younger children there is often cough and fever but no sputum production. Symptoms of general toxicity are more common with bacterial pneumonia.

The physical examination of a patient with pneumonia reveals one or several of the following signs: respiratory difficulty characterized by nasal flaring, rapid breathing, and intercostal, subcostal, and supraclavicular retractions; dullness to percussion in the involved area of the lung; and coarse breath sounds and fine rales on auscultation over the involved lung. The white blood cell count is usually elevated in bacterial pneumonia, but may be normal in viral and *Mycoplasma pneumoniae* pneumonias. A chest radiograph is very useful in making the diagnosis of pneumonia and in localizing exactly the extent of the pulmonary involvement.

Since most pneumonia is due to *Pneumococcus,* the most commonly used therapeutic agent is penicillin.

TUBERCULOSIS

Tuberculosis, which is produced by *Mycobacterium tuberculosis,* is still an important disease in the United States. World-wide it is one of the major causes of morbidity and mortality.

When a person comes in contact with *Mycobacterium tuberculosis* for the first time he may acquire primary tuberculosis, which is often a childhood problem. Following primary exposure to tuberculosis through the respiratory tract, the patient often develops a lung lesion associated with enlargement of intrathoracic lymph nodes; both of these findings are easily demonstrable on a chest radiograph. Most often the lesion stays localized within the lung producing a pneumonia, but occasionally there is spread throughout the body producing the so-called miliary tuberculosis and/or tuberculous meningitis.

Secondary or adult type of tuberculosis is usually a chronic, slowly progressing lesion at the upper tip of the lung; it is seldom a problem in childhood.

Tuberculosis may also enter the body through nonrespiratory routes such as the gastrointestinal tract, but nonrespiratory exposure is extremely rare in the United States because of the standards placed on dairy cows, which are the most common transmitters of nonrespiratory tuberculosis.

Tuberculin skin tests (see Chapter 8) are useful surveillance mechanisms against tuberculosis. When the tuberculin skin test becomes positive either because of exposure to *Mycobacterium tuberculosis* or BCG vaccine the periodic radiograph of the chest becomes the surveillance mechanism. Surveillance against tuberculosis is important to uncover epidemiologic foci since effective drug therapy is available. Children and adolescents who are found to have a positive tuberculin skin test without other evidence of disease are now usually treated prophylactically with drugs such as isoniazid.

Chapter 13
INFECTIOUS DISEASES

Infectious diseases are those diseases caused by infectious microorganisms—bacteria, viruses, spirochetes, fungi, and parasites. Some infectious diseases, such as measles or mumps, are communicable or contagious; that is, they spread from person to person. Others are not contagious since they do not spread from person to person but are spread by other ways (for example, through animal vectors).

In general, during the course of an infectious disease the patient passes through several stages. The *incubation* period is the time elapsed from the time of exposure to a particular agent to the time of onset of early clinical disease; this is a noncontagious period. The *prodromal* period is the early clinical phase, when the affected person has nonspecific symptoms such as runny nose, malaise, or fever; this is usually a very contagious period.

Because of the importance infectious diseases occupy in the practice of pediatrics, the pediatric nurse practitioner should be familiar both with general immunologic concepts and with some common infectious diseases.

BASIC IMMUNOLOGY

Principles of basic immunology are useful in understanding the body response not only to infection and immunologic deficiency diseases, but also to allergic and autoimmune diseases.

Antibody formation and phagocytosis are the two major mechanisms with which the body handles the intrusion of foreign substances. Foreign substances, whether bacterial, viral, or others, when introduced into the body, produce a response after a suitable interval. These foreign substances are referred to as antigens and the response of the body to the presence of an antigen is the production of antibodies. Microorganisms contain antigens and, when introduced into the body for the first time, trigger not only phagocytosis, which is the capture and killing of invading organisms, but also the production of antibodies. Should the person come in contact with the same microorganism again, the presence of antibodies formed in the first encounter with that antigen will enhance phagocytosis—thus the successful handling of that particular antigen.

The induction of antibody formation is the rationale behind immunization. A small dose of a specific antigen is purposely introduced into the body in order to elicit antibodies against that antigen. This process enables the body to fight that specific antigen successfully in future encounters with it. Once the body has produced antibodies to a foreign substance, either through a previous illness or through immunization, the body handles the invading organism (antigen) better in future encounters because the antibody response is extremely prompt. This anamnestic or booster response explains why three DPT injections are given initially, but only one booster injection is needed years later.

Although antibody formation should function as a defense mechanism of the body against harmful or potentially harmful agents, in allergic diseases such as hay fever or penicillin allergy, antibody formation is triggered by an otherwise harmless substance. After antibodies are present, future encounters with the antigen not only increase antibody formation but also produce a reaction in which histamine and other substances are released that are responsible for the allergic symptoms. Autoimmune diseases such as lupus erythematosus or rheumatoid arthritis are not well understood but it seems that the immunologic system of the host ceases to recognize certain tissues as its own, and antibody production against these tissues is induced.

The immunologic system is highly complex and not fully understood. Currently the immunologic system is divided into two functional components —the phagocytic cells and the cells of the lymphoid tissue with immunologic competence. The phagocytes are responsible for the engulfing and killing of invading microorganisms, a process which is enhanced by antibodies. The lymphoid tissues are further subdivided into (1) lymphocytes and thymus (T-cells), which are essential for cellular immunity, and (2) plasma cells (B-cells), which are responsible for humoral immunity.

The production of antibodies is often called humoral immunity, since antibodies are present in the blood, which is a fluid. When one administers gamma globulin as prophylaxis against disease the recipient is given antibodies. Plasma cells, which seem to come from lymphocytes, are responsible for the production of antibodies. Antibodies are plasma globulins (gamma globulin) and can be further subdivided into gamma G, M, A, D, and E. Gamma G accounts for approximately 90 percent of the adult gamma globulin. Since gamma G crosses the placenta, a normal newborn has close to the adult level of gamma globulin. However, transplacentally acquired gamma globulin from the mother disappears from the infant's system and he has to depend on his own production. Gamma globulin reaches its lowest level at about 3 months of age, a period called physiologic hypogammaglobulinemia, which is, as the name implies, entirely normal.

In addition to humoral immunity, the lymphocytes and thymus are responsible for cellular immunity. This type of immunity accounts for the resistance to certain infections, for delayed hypersensitivity such as reaction to the tuberculin skin test, and for graft rejection.

Diseases have been reported to be associated with the lack of one or several of the multiple components of the immunologic system; these diseases are called immunologic deficiency diseases. Children with immunologic deficiency diseases usually have frequent, severe infections that respond poorly to treatment (whereas the frequent respiratory infections of young children are usually self limited). Immunologic deficiency diseases are uncommon and are often hereditary, most frequently sex-linked recessive; that is, these diseases are very rare and even more so in females. In other words, before arriving at a diagnosis of immunologic deficiency, the patient needs to be evaluated by an expert in the field.

VIRAL DISEASES

Common cold. The common cold is an acute viral upper respiratory infection caused by one of several groups of respiratory viruses. Rhinoviruses, adenoviruses, influenza, and parainfluenza are the most significant.

The incubation period is less than 1 week and communicability is highest during the first 3 or 4 days of illness. Since a cold is transmitted by respiratory secretions, the incidence is higher during the winter, when indoor living increases. Since children have had little previous experiences with the different cold viruses, the incidence is higher during childhood. The average number of colds per year in preschool children is about eight; the average for adults is three colds per year.

A patient with a common cold has malaise, fever, runny nose, and sneezing lasting for 3 to 4 days. The management is entirely symptomatic and usually includes increased fluid intake to keep secretions loose; antipyretics such as aspirin to decrease fever; decongestants (vasoconstrictor nose drops such as phenylephrine or oral vasoconstrictors such as pseudoephedrine); and increased humidity. Either saline nose drops or a vaporizer humidifier is used to increase humidity. Some physicians prefer the use of vasoconstrictor nose drops but others feel that after 2 or 3 days these drops may produce rebound (a dry nasal plugging) and therefore prefer to use the oral vasoconstrictor agents or saline nose drops. Regardless of the methods used, keeping the secretions loose and the nasal and other respiratory channels open may prevent further complications such as ear infection. If, after 3 or 4 days, the patient develops an earache or becomes worse with increasing fever and sore throat, he has probably developed a bacterial superinfection and needs to be treated with antibiotics.

In order to make saline nose drops ¼ teaspoon of salt is diluted in 4 ounces of boiled water. Nasal suction with a soft rubber bulb syringe often helps infants who, of course, cannot blow their noses.

Rubeola (measles, hard measles). Measles is a highly communicable disease caused by a respiratory virus that spreads from person to person by droplet infection. Respiratory secretions or articles freshly soiled with respiratory secretions are the means of spread. The incubation period is usually 10 to 12 days. Measles is communicable from about 4 days before the appearance of the rash to 5 days after the rash appears.

Clinically, there is a prodromal period that includes fever, cough, malaise, runny nose, Koplik's spots, and watery eyes. Koplik's spots are fine white spots on a faint red base that appear in the mucous membrane of the mouth most often opposite to the first upper molar. The prodromal period is followed after 3 to 5 days by a maculopapular rash that first appears on the face and behind the ears. The temperature is often elevated to 103° or 104° F during the first 3 days after the rash appears, and the patient feels and looks ill. Photophobia is common and although no harm will result from exposure to bright lights, the patient is more comfortable in dim light or wearing dark glasses. The white blood cell count characteristically shows leukopenia (a decrease) unless there is a bacterial superinfection.

Some complications of measles are caused by a bacterial superinfection as in the case of pneumonia or otitis media. Others, such as encephalitis, are caused by the measles virus itself. Encephalitis occurs only in about 1 out of 1,000 cases, but often results in brain damage. Viral pneumonitis may also occur but is rare. Treatment for measles is only supportive with aspirin for fever or malaise and reassurance to the parents. Soon after exposure, measles can be prevented or at least modified with the administration of gamma globulin. Measles can also be prevented with measles or rubeola vaccine before exposure to the disease (see Chapter 8). Exposed children who have not had clinical measles and have not been immunized should receive gamma globulin to prevent or modify the disease.

Rubella (German measles, three-day measles). German measles is a mild communicable disease. It is not as contagious as rubeola and tends to occur in epidemics. It is caused by a respiratory virus and therefore is transmitted by respiratory droplets.

The incubation period lasts approximately 2 to 3 weeks. It is contagious from about 3 days before the rash appears to about 3 days after the appearance of the rash. However, newborn infants who contacted rubella in utero, the so-called "rubella babies," often shed the virus in the urine for up to 1½ years after birth and are therefore contagious as long as they shed the virus.

Clinically, rubella in children and adults is characterized by a prodromal period of malaise, mild temperature elevation (101° F), and enlarged tender postero-occipital lymph nodes. This is followed by a maculopapular rash, which starts on the face and back of the neck and spreads to the rest of the body. The white blood cell count, as in measles, is usually decreased.

Although encephalitis may occur in rubella, it is extremely rare and there are virtually no complications of rubella in childhood. The most significant complications are those occurring in pregnant women who have rubella. At least 20 percent of women who develop rubella during the first trimester of pregnancy deliver a "rubella baby" with one or all of the following: cataracts, congenital heart disease, deafness, mental retardation, and microcephaly.

The treatment of rubella is only supportive. Soon after exposure, gamma globulin prevents the manifestation of clinical disease. Since the disease is mild and without complications except in pregnancy, gamma globulin is recommended only for women exposed to rubella in early pregnancy. However, the value of gamma globulin in the prevention of the "rubella baby" is debatable. Rubella can be prevented if rubella vaccine is administered before exposure to the disease.

Roseola infantum (exanthema subitum). Roseola is probably caused by a respiratory virus, but the virus has never been isolated. The incubation period is estimated to be 1 to 2 weeks. The degree of communicability is not known, but the disease occurs in children between the ages of 6 months and 3 years.

Clinically, roseola is characterized by a high sustained or spiking fever lasting 3 to 5 days. A faint rash appears after the crisis occurs and the fever disappears. The white count is decreased as in measles. The diagnosis is difficult until the rash appears. However, the child does not look ill except that he is febrile.

The major complication of roseola is convulsion during the febrile period. No treatment is known except for supportive care to reduce the fever. Gamma globulin has no effect on this illness, and no vaccine is available. The pediatric nurse practitioner must often support the concerned family until the rash appears.

Erythema infectiosum (Fifth disease). Erythema infectiosum is probably caused by a respiratory virus, but the virus has never been isolated. The incubation period seems to be from 1 to 2 weeks. The disease occurs in families and in small epidemics but transmission, although probably through respiratory secretions, is not well understood. The disease occurs more often in children rather than in infants or adults.

Clinically, it is a mild, often afebrile illness in which the first signs are flushed cheeks and a rash. The rash is maculopapuloerythematous, which appears first on the cheeks. After 24 hours the rash occurs on the extensor surface of the extremities and finally on the trunk and flexor surfaces of the extremities. The rash may last from 2 days to 2 weeks. The white blood cell count is usually normal.

While no treatment is available, the illness is totally benign and without complications.

Varicella (chickenpox). Chickenpox is a highly communicable disease caused by a respiratory virus which spreads from person to person by droplets of respiratory secretions. The incubation period is approximately 13 to 17 days. The period of communicability is from 1 day before the onset of the rash to 7 days after onset.

Clinically, a patient with varicella manifests fever for 1 or 2 days prior to the appearance of a maculopapulovesicular rash. The rash appears in 2 to 6 crops. Each lesion starts as a clear fluid vesicle on a red base, which is called "tear drop." Subsequently the clear fluid becomes a papule with a crust. Leukopenia (decreased white blood cell count) is usually a finding in early chickenpox; however, the white blood cell count may rise if there is extensive secondary infection of the vesicles caused by scratching.

The most common complication of chickenpox is skin infection caused by scratching. Viral pneumonia with chickenpox, although severe if it occurs, is rare. Encephalitis is also a rare complication of chickenpox, but if it occurs it usually results in brain damage.

No treatment is available except symptomatic treatment for the fever and itching. Itching can be relieved with calamine lotion on the lesions, starch baths, or administration of oral antipruritic medication. The value of gamma globulin in chickenpox is very questionable. No vaccine is available.

Mumps (epidemic parotitis). Mumps is caused by a virus and is not as contagious as measles or chickenpox. It is spread by the saliva of affected persons. The incubation period lasts approximately 18 days but it can be as long as 4 weeks. The period of communicability is from 7 days before the onset of the parotid swelling until the swelling disappears approximately 9 days later.

Clinically a prodromal period of malaise and fever that lasts from 1 to 2 days is followed by salivary gland swelling. Most often the parotid gland at the angle of the jaw is involved, but the submaxillary salivary glands may be involved. When the parotid gland is swollen it is often difficult to differentiate it from swelling of the cervical lymph nodes; however, parotid swelling usually involves the angle of the jaw extending up to the area in front of the ear. The white cell count is usually normal or decreased in mumps. Mumps meningoencephalitis, as diagnosed by examination of the cerebrospinal fluid, occurs in as many as 70 percent of all cases but is extremely benign. Brain damage is extremely rare. Clinical symptoms of meningoencephalitis such as headache, vomiting, and stiff neck occur in only 25 percent of the cases of mumps and may even precede parotitis by 2 to 5 days. Numerous other organs such as testicles, ovaries, pancreas, kidneys, and ears may be affected in mumps. Testicular involvement almost never occurs before puberty; after puberty testicular involvement occurs in approximately 30 percent of the cases. In half of these cases (15 percent of all cases) the involvement is bilateral and complete sterility can occur. However, complete sterility occurs only in 2 to 3 percent of all cases of mumps in postpubertal males. Hearing nerve involvement from mumps is a frequent cause of hearing loss.

No treatment is available for mumps other than supportive or symptomatic care. Gamma globulin is of no value. However, the mumps vaccine currently available is very effective if given before exposure. At present, it is still not known how long immunity lasts after the vaccine. Since mumps in childhood is fairly benign, the vaccine is recommended only for children 10 years of age or older who have not had the disease because the incidence of other complications such as testicular or ovarian involvement is greater for these children.

Viral hepatitis. Viral hepatitis includes two separate entities that are caused by two seemingly different viruses, the infectious hepatitis virus and the serum hepatitis virus.

Clinically they both produce fever, malaise, chills, vomiting, headache, and jaundice. Jaundice appears 2 to 5 days after the fever and lasts for several weeks. However, epidemiologically, the two viruses are different. Infectious hepatitis is transmitted both orally or ano-orally and parenterally by needles or blood transfusion. Serum hepatitis is almost always transmitted parenterally. The incubation period is from 2 to 6 weeks for infectious hepatitis and from 2 to 6 months for serum hepatitis.

Impairment of liver function by viral hepatitis is temporary in most patients and the liver recuperates completely. However, in a few patients the liver is permanently damaged with subsequent development of cirrhosis. Fortunately, posthepatitis cirrhosis is less common in children than in adults.

No treatment for viral hepatitis is available except for a high protein, low fat diet with adequate carbohydrate intake and bed rest, which does not have to be necessarily strict especially for children. Gamma globulin is of value in decreasing the severity of the disease and in preventing liver damage when given soon after exposure. The doses of gamma globulin required in infectious and in serum hepatitis are different, and the value of gamma globulin is greater in infectious hepatitis. It is currently recommended that household contacts receive gamma globulin when infectious hepatitis is diagnosed in a member of the household.

Herpes simplex. Herpes simplex virus causes common "cold sores" or "fever blisters." Although most initial infections with this virus are asymptomatic, herpes simplex virus can produce an acute inflammation of the mouth, female genitalia, or eyes.

The clinical manifestation of acute infection often is gingivostomatitis (inflammation of oral mucosa and gums), which is most common between the ages of 1 and 3 years. The gums become red and swollen, and vesicles, which soon become ulcers, appear in the oral mucosa. Fever is usually associated with the gingivostomatitis.

No specific treatment is known, but since the intake of food is painful, topical astringents such as glyoxide and anesthetic agents such as viscous xylocaine are of value. Occasionally, pain is so severe that even liquids are refused and intravenous hydration may be required.

The prognosis is excellent but severe encephalitis may result in rare cases, especially in newborns and debilitated infants. Recurrent infection ("cold sores" and "fever blisters") may occur subsequent to the acute infection.

Infectious mononucleosis. Infectious mononucleosis is an infectious, not very contagious, disease probably caused by the Ebstein-Barr (EB) virus.

Clinically, it is characterized by fever, malaise, sore throat often with exudate, enlarged lymph nodes, and splenomegaly. In some cases there may be liver enlargement, jaundice, and a rash. The total white count is normal but the differential count usually shows characteristically large, atypical lymphocytes. The diagnosis is made by a blood test called heterophile agglutination test or, more recently, by the slide "Mono Spot" test.

The illness persists 2 to 6 weeks. The treatment is only symptomatic. Bed rest is of no proved value and the child's feelings should dictate his level of activity. However, vigorous physical exercise is contraindicated while splenomegaly persists.

Influenza. Influenza is an acute respiratory viral disease that occurs in epidemics. Clinically, its manifestations are fever, malaise, aching muscles, headache, and coughing. The white blood cell count is usually normal unless there are complications.

The complications are usually bacterial such as otitis media and pneumonia and, very rarely, viral encephalitis.

Treatment is only symptomatic unless complications occur. A vaccine is available but its use is primarily recommended for chronically ill children such as those with cystic fibrosis.

BACTERIAL DISEASES

Streptococcal diseases. Group A beta hemolytic *Streptococcus* is the common *Streptococcus* producing "strep throat."

Infection with group A beta hemolytic *Streptococcus* usually produces high fever. The throat is red with white exudate particularly when the disease occurs in middle childhood. In early childhood the disease is more insidious and is characterized by runny nose, nonexudative tonsillitis, or otitis media.

Scarlet fever is also a common manifestation of streptococcal disease in middle childhood. The rash is caused by an erythrogenic toxin produced by specific streptococci. Scarlet fever rash occurs only if a person who has no protection against the toxin is infected with a toxin-producing *Streptococcus.* Since the erythrogenic toxin is the same in all streptococci that produce it, scarlet fever or scarlatina rash occurs only once. The eruption is a diffuse, finely papular, bright red erythema, which blanches on pressure. Unlike measles, it starts at the base of the neck, axillae, and groin, and spreads to the trunk and extremities. The face is flushed with circumoral (around the mouth) pallor but true rash or exanthem does not occur in the face. In the flexure of the elbow the rash forms red lines, called Pastia's lines, that do not blanch.

In acute streptococcal disease the white blood cell count is usually elevated and there is a predominance of polymophonuclear leukocytes. Many of these leukocytes are immature (the so-called shift to the left—that is, a greater number of immature polymorphonuclear leukocytes in the peripheral blood).

The complications of streptococcal disease include purulent diseases, such as cervical adenitis or mastoiditis, and nonpurulent complications, such as rheumatic fever (see Chapter 14) and nephritis (see Chapter 16). Nonpurulent complications of streptococcal disease are common in middle and late childhood but are rare in early childhood.

The drug of choice against *Streptococcus* is penicillin administered for 10 days in order to prevent complications such as rheumatic fever. Erythromycin is the second drug of choice and is used for persons sensitive to penicillin.

Pertussis (whooping cough). Whooping cough is caused by a bacterium called *Bordetella pertussis,* which is transmitted by respiratory droplets. The incubation period lasts about 10 days and the disease is communicable. Communicability usually is from 1 week before the onset of paroxysmal coughing to 3 weeks after onset.

Clinically, pertussis consists of three stages: a cold-like stage called the catarrhal period, which lasts 2 weeks; a severe coughing stage called the paroxysmal period, which lasts 2 weeks, and finally a convalescent state lasting 2 weeks.

Characteristically, the white blood cell count is elevated up to 20,000 to 30,000 per cu mm with a predominance of small lymphocytes. Cultures in special media are required for the definitive diagnosis.

Most of the morbidity and mortality in pertussis occur during the first year of life as a result of pulmonary complications, such as pneumonia, atelectasis, and bronchiectasis, and to central nervous system damage that is probably secondary to anoxia. Because of the high incidence of complications in infants and because infants are not protected against pertussis transplacentally, immunization against pertussis is started early in life (see Chapter 8).

The drug of choice at present is erythromycin. Pertussis hyperimmune globulin is of value in young infants who are exposed to pertussis and who have not been protected by vaccination. Vaccination against pertussis is usually administered as diphtheria-pertussis-tetanus (DPT) to infants. If given before exposure, DPT prevents the disease.

Chapter 14

THE CARDIOVASCULAR SYSTEM

Cardiovascular evaluation is an integral part of the physical examination in infants and children. The pediatric nurse practitioner should be concerned primarily with detecting cardiovascular anomalies during health supervision and with suspecting rheumatic fever in a child with an acute illness.

CONGENITAL ANOMALIES

Identification of congenital heart disease is the primary purpose of cardiovascular screening in infancy and early childhood.

The incidence of congenital heart anomalies is approximately 5 per 1,000 live births. The three most common diseases, which account for 50 percent of all congenital heart defects in children, are ventricular septal heart defects, patent ductus arteriosus, and tetralogy of Fallot. In school-age children, however, atrial septal defect and pulmonary and aortic stenosis are the more prevalent diagnoses. Since one fourth to one third of all deaths from congenital heart disease occur in the first month of life, it is of utmost importance to evaluate the hearts of newborns and infants carefully.

The best screening method for such evaluation is physical examination including blood pressure, evaluation of femoral pulses, and examination of the heart proper. Femoral pulses are obtained by palpating in the middle upper thigh immediately under the fold of the groin. Absence of femoral pulses suggests coarctation of the aorta.

The three major clinical methods to determine blood pressure are (1) auscultatory, which is familiar to most nurses; (2) palpatory, which gives only systolic blood pressure and is also well known to most nurses; and (3) flush, which is probably not as widely used among nurses but it is used frequently in infants and young children because of difficulties with other methods. To obtain a flush blood pressure, a blood pressure cuff is applied to the wrist or ankle. The part of the extremity distal to the cuff is compressed by wrapping, the cuff is compressed to 200 mm of pressure, and the wrapping is removed. The pressure in the cuff is then released slowly until the blanched part of the extremity flushes. Flush pressure is approximately midway between systolic and diastolic blood pressure.

Examination of the heart proper consists of observing the left side of the chest for unusual prominence and for precordial activity, which may be related to heart size. The point of maximal impulse, which indicates the point where the apex of the heart hits the chest wall, can also be observed and palpated and is indicative of heart size. Thrills, which are vibratory sensations due to abnormal turbulence of blood in the heart, are always abnormal (see Chapter 3).

On auscultation of the heart one first determines the type of rhythm (see Chapter 3) and then listens for the presence or absence of murmurs. If murmurs are present, it is important for the examiner to differentiate between normal (functional or innocent) and abnormal (organic) murmurs. Functional murmurs do not indicate an abnormality in the heart and are present in more than half of all children at some time in their life. In the newborn, functional systolic murmurs are often heard to the left of the sternum in the third and fourth interspace. In older children soft, and at times musical or squeaky midsystolic functional murmurs are heard along the left side of the sternum and at the base of the heart. They are generally heard at the pulmonary valve focus, which is at the second left intercostal space (see Chapter 3). These murmurs may become less audible or disappear when the patient exercises or sits up. Functional murmurs are always systolic, that is, they are heard after the first heart sound. Functional murmurs are more frequently present when the child has an acute febrile illness.

RHEUMATIC FEVER

Rheumatic fever often affects the heart and is a complication of an untreated or inadequately treated streptococcal disease. The prevalence of rheumatic heart disease among school children is about 1 per 1,000 children.

Abnormal heart murmurs, fever, rash, nodules under the skin, and migratory joint swelling are among the most frequent clinical signs associated with rheumatic fever. However, the diagnosis of rheumatic fever is difficult and is not within the scope of this book.

It is important to realize that many children who are said to have had rheumatic fever but without good evidence for the diagnosis may become crippled because of family overprotection. Once a child has had rheumatic fever and has recovered from the acute illness, his activities should not be limited, except if there is severe permanent heart damage. The child should, however, be on prophylactic penicillin at least through young adulthood to prevent future heart damage. The usual prophylactic dose of penicillin is 250 mg morning and night orally. If there is poor cooperation in taking the drug regularly, one dose of 1.2 million units of benzathine penicillin per month is equally effective.

FAINTING

Fainting, or syncope, is a sudden loss of consciousness, which may have numerous and varied causes. Most fainting is the result of vasodepressor syncope (simple fainting). However, the cause may be cardiac as in aortic stenosis, metabolic as in hypoglycemia, epileptic as in convulsive disorder, or emotional as in hyperventilation or in breath-holding spells.

An etiologic diagnosis is important in order to institute proper management. The most common fainting episodes in older children and adolescents are simple fainting or vasodepressor attacks. They are often precipitated by sudden danger, real or imaginary, such as the sight of blood. When the pediatric nurse practitioner cannot make a diagnosis of simple fainting, the patient needs further evaluation to determine the cause.

In simple fainting (vasodepressor syncope) the patient develops a reflex vasodilation, which temporarily decreases the blood supply to the brain. Clinically, the patient becomes pale and sweaty, may have a few twitches of the facial and arm muscles, and eventually loses consciousness.

As soon as the patient lies down, adequate circulation to the brain is restored and consciousness is regained. Therefore, the most effective treatment of simple fainting spells is to place the patient in a recumbent position.

Chapter 15

THE DIGESTIVE SYSTEM

The pediatric nurse practitioner often deals with problems of the digestive system including malocclusion, anorexia in toddlers, abdominal pain, vomiting, diarrhea, and constipation with or without encopresis.

TEETH

Dental cavities. During the examination of the mouth, observation of the teeth is often neglected by the examiner who is not a dentist. However, approximately half of all 2-year-old children have at least one cavity; this incidence increases to 80 percent in children older than 6 years of age.

Although genetic factors seem to be important in the resistance to cavities, health education can be helpful, since proper fluoridation of water, adequate diet, and proper oral hygiene will reduce the incidence of dental caries.

A concentration of fluoride in the drinking water of 1 part per million will significantly decrease cavities. Should the community water not be naturally fluoridated, artificial fluoridation to a concentration of 1 part per million is recommended. Where adequate fluoridation of drinking water cannot be accomplished, topical fluoride treatment by a dental professional as well as ingestion of vitamins with fluoride is beneficial.

In order to prevent dental cavities the consumption of sweets between meals should be discouraged. Health professionals should discuss the importance of oral hygiene in the prevention of cavities. The frequency of brushing of the teeth should coincide with the frequency of eating and the type of food ingested.

Malocclusion. Proper occlusion is necessary for proper mastication or chewing. When dental malocclusion or abnormal opposition of the upper and lower teeth is evident, the nurse practitioner should suggest referral to an orthodontist.

Thumb-sucking is often blamed for malocclusion; however, it does not produce malocclusion unless it persists after the age of 5 or 6 years when the permanent incisors first erupt. Thumb-sucking is often the result of insecurity; the cause of the child's insecurity should be sought and treated rather than the habit itself. The parents should be encouraged not to attempt to correct the habit directly but rather to try to correct the emotional problem behind it.

COLIC

Infantile colic refers to recurrent sharp abdominal pain associated with severe crying occurring in infants under 3 months of age.

An infant suffering from colic usually cries suddenly and loudly, his face flushes, his abdomen becomes distended and tense, and he draws up his legs although he may momentarily extend them. The attack may persist for several hours and frequently recurs at the same time of the day.

Although numerous causes such as hunger, air-swallowing, overfeeding, and maternal insecurity are associated with infantile colic, and certain infants seem more susceptible to colic than others, the etiology of infantile colic is not well understood.

Reassurance to the parents is always in order, since the condition almost never persists after 3 months of age. Sedation for some infants with severe attacks is recommended by some physicians.

ANOREXIA IN THE TODDLER

As mentioned in Chapter 5, the rate of weight gain decreases in the second year of life, and there is a normal decrease in appetite.

Parents need to be reassurred of the fact that this decrease in weight gain is normal. It should also be remembered that during this same time children are going through a period of psychologic negativism during which they respond with "no" to most commands. Therefore, children should not be nagged to eat but provided with a balanced diet and allowed to feed themselves. Eating between meals may be discouraged so that the child will have more appetite for three well-balanced meals. On the other hand, some children do better with frequent small meals; they should be offered snacks consisting of fruit juices, crackers, cheese, and other healthful foods rather than cookies and candies.

ABDOMINAL PAIN

Approximately 10 percent of school-age children suffer recurrent abdominal pain. It is slightly more common in girls than in boys. There are many causes of abdominal pain in children but they can be grouped into organic and nonorganic.

Organic abdominal pain is caused by pathology in one of the several intra-abdominal organ systems. The child may have appendicitis, Meckel's diverticulitis, malrotation, volvulus, intussusception, or constipation.

In the genitourinary system conditions such as obstructive uropathy, urinary tract infection, dysmenorrhea, or a torsion of an ovary may produce abdominal pain. Mesenteric lymphadenitis, crisis of sickle cell anemia, and pneumonia may also produce abdominal pain in children.

Although organic causes of abdominal pain must be carefully considered, psychogenic factors are responsible for most of the recurrent abdominal pain in children. Both the history and the physical examination are useful in differentiating organic from psychogenic pain. The pain in psychogenic abdominal pain is usually epigastric (above the umbilicus) or periumbilical. Its character and intensity can be easily mistaken for an organic problem such as early appendicitis. However, the pain caused by appendicitis or Meckel's diverticulitis usually increases in severity during a 24-hour period with vomiting, absence of bowel sounds in auscultation of the abdomen, and an increase in the white blood cell count.

The history of the chronic recurrent character of the pain. becomes important because an acute episode of either appendicitis or Meckel's diverticulitis usually ends in bowel perforation unless surgery is done within 24 to 48 hours. Therefore, if the child has a history of similar episodes of recurrent pain, the pain is probably psychogenic. Abdominal pain is even more likely to be psychogenic in origin when the parents seem to be anxious and overprotective. If the pain is psychogenic the practitioner should talk to the family and should set up subsequent visits to attempt to discover and handle the disturbing problem for the child. However, the nurse practitioner should always remember that organic disease may occur in children who also have psychogenic pain; therefore, a careful physical evaluation of the patient should not be omitted.

VOMITING AND DIARRHEA

Regurgitation of some portion of a feeding in young infants is extremely common and it should be ignored if the child is gaining weight well and seems healthy otherwise.

An acute episode of vomiting and diarrhea frequently is caused either by overeating or by an acute infection (often considered viral) of the gastrointestinal tract. However, there are many other causes of vomiting and diarrhea.

Besides treating the underlying disease, the most important therapeutic measure that should be undertaken is dietary restriction (see dehydration in Chapter 11).

Parents should be instructed to either call or return to the health care facility if the child does not show improvement 24 hours after measures for rehydration are initiated. The child should also return if the symptoms are unusually serious (especially if the patient is very young), if there is high or prolonged fever, if the urine output diminishes greatly, or if there is blood in the stool. An acute onset of severe abdominal pain and currant jelly–like stool suggest intussusception or telescoping of one part of the intestine into another. This is often a complication of acute gastroenteritis.

CONSTIPATION AND ENCOPRESIS

Constipation is discussed with encopresis because encopresis is often the end result of severe prolonged constipation. Encopresis is fecal soiling after the age of bowel training, and, as expected, is extremely disruptive to the child's social adjustment.

Encopresis, which occurs in 1 to 2 percent of school-age children, is usually an "overflow" incontinence in patients with severe constipation caused by psychologic problems.

Since constipation in children is often a symbolic manifestation of the inability to express their feelings, the nurse practitioner needs to work with the family of a patient with constipation with or without encopresis in order that the child may learn to express his feelings. Physically, the child should be evaluated for organic causes of constipation such as anal fissure or Hirschsprung's disease.

Bowel softeners and suppositories at regular intervals to allow regular bowel movements are often of help when the child is so severely constipated as to have encopresis. This treatment will often render the child free of encopresis while the nurse practitioner has time to deal with the psychologic problem. If constipation and encopresis do not subside more expert psychologic help needs to be obtained.

HERNIAS

Although treatment of hernias is surgical, it is within the responsibility of the pediatrician or the nurse practitioner to diagnose them. Umbilical, inguinal, and femoral hernias are the most common hernias in children.

Umbilical hernias, as the name suggests, are located at the navel or umbilical scar. If the defect in the abdominal wall is less than 2.5 cm in diameter no treatment is necessary until the child is 4 to 5 years of age. Taping, a common popular treatment, does not help and may introduce infection. Most umbilical hernias disappear by themselves. Rarely they become incarcerated (irreducible) or strangulated (with compromised circulation). Should umbilical hernias become incarcerated or strangulated they need to be treated by surgery immediately. Otherwise, they should be repaired if they have not disappeared by 5 years of age.

Inguinal hernia needs to be differentiated from hydrocele, which is an accumulation of fluid between the covers of the testicle and spermatic cord. Hydroceles are usually oval, fluctuant, and unlike hernias, are translucent to light. They are common in newborn infants and often disappear by themselves. Hydroceles, when not associated with a hernia, require no treatment if they do not communicate with the peritoneal cavity. If they do communicate the treatment is the same as for inguinal hernias.

Femoral hernias and the more common inguinal hernias are located in the groin. The former are located in the middle upper thigh under the groin; the latter occur in the groin in the inguinal canal and sometimes go into the scrotum. Both of these hernias need to be repaired since they do not go away by themselves, and they tend to incarcerate and strangulate easily.

Chapter 16

THE GENITOURINARY SYSTEM

Several diseases of the genitourinary system, such as urinary tract infection, nephritis, nephrosis, enuresis, and undescended testicles, should be of interest to the pediatric nurse practitioner.

URINARY TRACT INFECTION

Urinary tract infection is a common acute illness for which children are brought for medical help. Although urinary tract infection is suspected in a child with fever, back pain, and dysuria (painful urination), these classical symptoms may be absent. Urinary tract infection should be suspected in patients with fever without obvious cause. The diagnosis is made by examination of the urine in which protein (albumin), bacteria, and casts may be found. Pyuria, which is an excess amount of white blood cells in the urine, may also occur. The urine, especially in girls, should be collected by the midstream clean catch method in order to prevent contamination with the bacteria and white cells that are present in other secretions.

The diagnosis of urinary tract infection is confirmed by urine culture. Most urinary infections are caused by intestinal bacteria (gram negative bacilli), but other organisms may also cause it. Usually a culture of greater than 100,000 or 10^6 organisms per cu mm indicates bacteriuria (abnormal presence of bacteria in the urine); below 100,000 per cu mm but greater than 1,000 is of questionable significance and the culture should be repeated; if below 1,000 per cu mm, the culture is considered negative.

Because gram negative bacilli usually cause urinary infection, a sulfonamide, such as sulfisoxasole is the drug of choice.

It is extremely important to obtain urine for urinalysis and urine culture after treatment in order to prevent chronic urinary infection caused by incomplete eradication of the infection. It is also important that urologic tests such as intravenous pyelogram, voiding cystourethrogram, and possibly cystoscopy be done after the first infection in a boy and after the second infection in a girl. These investigations are done to detect any abnormality that might be responsible for obstruction of the urinary drainage. Urologic investigations are done after the first infection in boys rather than after the second, because the incidence of obstructive uropathy in boys with urinary tract infection is higher than in girls. Careful evaluation and follow-up of a patient with urinary tract infection is essential, since chronic or recurrent asymptomatic infection may lead to severe irreversible kidney damage.

NEPHRITIS (GLOMERULONEPHRITIS)

Acute glomerulonephritis seems to be a nonsuppurative reaction to streptococcal infection due to an allergic response to a few specific strains of streptococci.

Nephritis is rare under the age of 3 years. The patient usually presents with the complaint of a "smoky or cloudy urine" and in some cases the eyes are puffy because of retention of fluid (edema). Physical examination usually reveals hypertension.

Laboratory examination of the urine reveals proteinuria, hematuria, and casts, the most diagnostic of which are red blood cell casts or casts with red cells inside. Chemical examination of the blood usually reveals elevated blood urea nitrogen levels.

Although the prognosis of acute glomerulonephritis is good, from 1 to 2 percent of the patients die because of cardiac failure, kidney failure, or central nervous system damage secondary to the hypertension. Of those that survive about 2 percent will develop chronic glomerulonephritis with progressive slow deterioration of kidney function.

The treatment of acute glomerulonephritis is mostly supportive—treatment of the cardiac failure and of the hypertension as necessary.

NEPHROSIS (NEPHROTIC SYNDROME)

Nephrosis is a disease of unknown etiology. It occurs in children 2 to 5 years old and is characterized by edema, proteinuria, decrease in serum protein levels, and increase in serum cholesterol. A transient elevation of the blood pressure and often of the blood urea nitrogen level may be present; however, both should be worrisome signs of more serious kidney damage such as chronic glomerulonephritis presenting as a nephrosis. The treatment is nonspecific, but steroids and immunosuppressive agents are often used. The prognosis is at best guarded since most patients will recover from the first episode but, of these, many will continue to have recurrent exacerbations with slow deterioration of kidney function.

ORTHOSTATIC ALBUMINURIA

Orthostatic albuminuria is a benign condition in which the patient shows no other urinary findings except the presence of an abnormal amount of protein in the urine.

As many as 5 percent of all children have orthostatic albuminuria. The cause is not well determined, but it seems to be due to alteration in the renal arterial circulation during the erect or standing position. Therefore, the first morning urine does not have an abnormal amount of protein. The prognosis is excellent, although some investigators claim that some of these patients with orthostatic albuminuria have an underlying, more serious pathology such as lupus erythematosus.

ENURESIS

Enuresis or bed-wetting is found in as many as 15 to 20 percent of school-age children, but there is a definite male predominance.

A urinalysis should always be done and a subsequent urologic work-up should be obtained if the urinalysis is abnormal or if the enuresis persists. In a small percentage of cases an underlying organic cause may be present, but in the great majority of cases the cause is psychogenic.

The most frequent psychopathology associated with enuresis is repressed aggression. Thus, in counseling a family with an enuretic child, a psycho-analytic therapist will first establish a relationship with the child and then will try to uncover the reasons why the child's aggressiveness is stimulated and repressed and will allow the child to ventilate his feelings. A behaviorist therapist will design a program of positive reinforcements to reward the child every day he wakes up dry. Regardless of the orientation of the therapist it is important to stop the probable fight going on between the child and his mother concerning his enuresis. Several practical suggestions may be helpful, such as buying waterproof pads to be placed on the child's bed to prevent wetting of the sheets and mattress and, therefore, diminishing this area of conflict. Also, no punishment should be inflicted. Other therapeutic measures tried are an alarm system to wake the child when he wets, bladder stretching exercises, and drugs to relax the bladder. Although none of the numerous therapeutic measures tried for enuresis are extremely successful, time cures most enuretic children.

UNDESCENDED TESTICLES

Cryptorchidism or undescended testicle in one or both sides is not an unusual finding in boys. The examiner needs to be sure that it is not confused with pseudocryptorchidism due to retraction of the testicle into the inguinal canal, which may occur when a child is afraid or upset. When the child has cryptorchidism he should be observed until 3 years of age, at which time referral should be made for appropriate medical or surgical treatment in order to prevent testicular damage caused by the higher intra-abdominal temperature.

DYSMENORRHEA

Dysmenorrhea, or painful, difficult menstruation, is a common problem among adolescent girls.

Dysmenorrhea is classified as primary and secondary. Primary dysmenorrhea is not associated with anatomic abnormalities, while secondary dysmenorrhea is due to an anatomic problem. Most adolescent dysmenorrhea is of the primary type.

Numerous drugs have been used in the treatment of dysmenorrhea. However, the treatment of primary dysmenorrhea should consist of counseling to ease tension and to change attitudes in order to decrease fear of menstruation, so that patients will better tolerate whatever discomfort they may have. In severe cases, referral to a gynecologist is sometimes necessary.

Chapter 17

THE ENDOCRINE SYSTEM

The endocrine organs are the pituitary, thyroid, parathyroid, and adrenal glands, the pancreas, ovaries, and testes. The principal conditions with which the pediatric nurse practitioner should be familiar are breast enlargement in boys, menstruation (see Chapter 16), diabetes mellitus, and growth failure.

PHYSIOLOGIC BREAST HYPERTROPHY

Physiologic breast hypertrophy, or physiologic gynecomastia, is a common condition in adolescent boys. It is characterized by slight enlargement of one or both breasts which, as with normal breast development in females, is often asymmetric.

The cause of this phenomenon is not well understood. It usually persists only a few months but it can last as long as a few years, although it rarely lasts longer than 2 years.

No treatment is necessary, but the patient, of course, needs to be reassured. Endocrinologic studies are seldom indicated if there are no other signs or symptoms of endocrinologic disease.

GROWTH FAILURE

Growth failure means lack of normal progress in physical growth of a particular child when he is compared with his peers. Ultimately growth is hormonally controlled and for this reason growth failure is included in the endocrine section of this book. In a child who is evaluated for growth failure it is of utmost importance to determine by frequent serial measurements whether he is indeed a child who is growing abnormally or a normal child who is at the extreme of the normal scale. Since growth failure may be caused by psychosocial, organic, or genetic causes, the patient most often needs a thorough and extensive evaluation.

Psychosocial causes for growth failure are poorly understood but are also the most frequent factors. As many as 75 percent of children with growth failure show evidence of disturbed interpersonal relationships at home, a fact which may or may not be associated with chronic underfeeding of the child.

There are many organic factors related to growth failure, although this type of growth failure does not occur as frequently as psychosocial growth failure. Some of these factors are congenital infection, defects in a major organ system, and genetic or constitutional factors. Defects of major organs include congenital heart disease, malabsorption, generalized skeletal defects, mental retardation, and defects of the urinary and endocrine systems, all of which may cause growth failure. Hereditary causes include detectable chromosomal errors as those occurring in mongolism. Delayed puberty and primordial dwarfism, although not caused by detectable chromosomal errors, can also be the cause of growth retardation on a hereditary or constitutional basis. Primordial dwarfism is a rare cause of growth failure in which the patient resembles a pituitary dwarf but does not lack, and does not respond to, growth hormone as the pituitary dwarf does.

DIABETES MELLITUS

Diabetes mellitus in its juvenile and adult forms is a disease produced by the malfunction of the pancreas, which either decreases or stops the production of insulin.

The adult form begins during adulthood and it is insidious in onset; the juvenile form begins during childhood or young adulthood and progresses rapidly so that children are usually brought for medical help within 3 months of the onset of diabetes.

The classic symptoms of early diabetes mellitus are frequency and increased amount of urine (polyuria), thirst and increased fluid intake (polydypsia), loss of weight, and increased appetite (polyphagia).

In general, juvenile diabetes mellitus is more severe and therefore more difficult to control than the adult type. In other words, diabetic children go into insulin reaction or diabetic coma more easily. Insulin reaction is extreme hypoglycemia, caused by an overdose of insulin for the caloric intake. Diabetic coma is extreme hyperglycemia or increased blood sugar together with acidosis caused by an increased production of acid metabolites due to an excessive burning of fat. The daily variation in the amount of physical activity of most children and the fact that older children and adolescents psychologically either fight or deny that they have diabetes make the management difficult.

Education of parents and children is extremely necessary for the adequate management of diabetes mellitus. The pediatric nurse practitioner needs to explain to the patient and his parents the need for insulin, the need for special diet, and the need to check the urine three times a day for sugar content. Children should be taught to recognize symptoms of hypoglycemia and should know how to abort further manifestations by consuming sugar orally. Although insulin doses need to be regulated by the physician, parents and adolescent patients should learn to make minor adjustments in insulin dosage when needed. There are numerous preparations available, some longer acting than others. During infection, as with a cold, the insulin requirement increases. It is important to stress that in our present state of knowledge parenteral insulin will always be necessary for diabetic patients.

The dietary management of juvenile diabetes varies somewhat depending on the preferences of the physician. Diet instructions for diabetic patients are best given by a dietitian together with a physician. In general the pediatric nurse practitioner needs to know that although some diets are unnecessarily rigid, the calories should not vary significantly from day to day if the patient's activity does not vary greatly. Caloric intake should not be excessive, and meals should be eaten at approximately the same time each day. Some physicians prefer for the carbohydrate content not to exceed 40 percent of the total caloric content of the diet and the protein to be about 20 percent of the total caloric content of the diet.

Urine determination for sugar can be best accomplished by Clini-Test tablets or Test-Tape, both of which come with a color chart and instructions. Because children are more severe diabetics and are more unstable, most physicians caring for diabetics recommend maintaining the urine sugar between 1 + and 2 +.

Diabetic emergencies. Diabetic emergencies are mainly either insulin reaction or diabetic coma. Without question the most important diabetic emergency is an insulin reaction—an extreme hypoglycemia caused by an excessive dose of insulin. Insulin reaction may damage the brain. Diabetic coma, or diabetic acidosis, usually does not damage the brain. When the examiner is not sure whether a child is having an insulin reaction or is in diabetic coma it is best to give him sugar, for example, 50 milliliters of 50 percent glucose intravenously, and observe the reaction. If he has a good response, this is followed by giving the patient sugar-containing fluid orally or intravenously depending on the situation. Glucagon, which releases sugar from the liver, may also be given intramuscularly in a dose of 1 ml. If the child responds, oral sugar should then be given.

The child in diabetic coma needs both insulin and fluid containing sugar administered intravenously because of the severity of the situation.

Chapter 18

THE MUSCULOSKELETAL SYSTEM

The pediatric nurse practitioner should be acquainted with several conditions of the musculoskeletal system such as malformation of the feet caused by intrauterine positions, pigeon toes, bowlegs, and congenital dislocation of the hip.

MALPOSITION OF THE FEET CAUSED BY INTRAUTERINE POSITION

The newborn usually has a position of comfort for his body in which the feet often adopt odd positions; many of these positions appear abnormal and sometimes suggest absence of muscles or bones.

However, as long as one is able to overcorrect the position (for example, turning the feet down and inward if they are up and outward), the only treatment needed is reassurance. Passive exercise done by manually overcorrecting the involved foot and active exercise by scratching the foot to elicit overcorrection may accelerate the eventual recovery.

PIGEON TOE

Pigeon toe or toeing-in is a frequent complaint. Metatarsus adductus, in which the forefoot points inward and the hind foot is normal, is one of the most common causes of pigeon toes. Inward tibial torsion and inward femoral torsion may also cause pigeon toe.

Inward tibial torsion and inward femoral torsion require no treatment, since growth will induce spontaneous correction. Metatarsus adductus should be treated early in order to avoid the need for prolonged and expensive further treatment. If treated early the feet need only to be forced outward by using orthopedic shoes or by reversing shoes (left shoe on right foot and right shoe on left foot), which in bilateral metatarsus adductus accomplishes in an inexpensive way the same result as with more costly orthopedic shoes. If there is no improvement the child should be referred to an orthopedic surgeon.

BOWLEGS

Bowlegs, a common condition in infancy, refers to an arching of the tibia usually associated with some internal tibial torsion.

Although several uncommon pathologic states such as rickets and Blount's disease may produce bowlegs, this condition usually is physiologic and will correct itself spontaneously. Parents need only reassurance. If bowing is severe or becomes more pronounced with growth, a single radiographic examination of the knee and lower leg is sometimes indicated to uncover possible pathologic states.

CONGENITAL DISLOCATION OF THE HIP

Congenital dislocation of the hip is an abnormality in which the acetabulum, or socket, of the hip that receives the head of the femur is too shallow and thus the femur becomes easily dislocated. The incidence is about 1 per 1,000 live births with a hereditary tendency. The condition occurs most commonly in girls.

Among the numerous physical and radiologic signs to diagnose congenital dislocation of the hip in infancy, one of the most useful early signs is Ortolani's maneuver. Ortolani's maneuver is performed by placing the infant on his back; thighs are flexed and the knees are then abducted passively until they nearly reach the examining table. If resistance is met at 60 to 70 degrees, dislocation of the hips is suspected. If the leg is completely dislocated at the hip, the affected leg will be shorter. When congenital dislocation of the hip is suspected, radiologic examination is indicated.

The prognosis is very good if the condition is diagnosed early. In such cases an orthopedic surgeon will only take measures to keep the femoral head inside the acetabulum, which will result in good formation of the acetabulum and therefore in a normal hip. Failure to recognize this disorder in early infancy usually necessitates prolonged and costly treatment, which does not always prevent permanent disability.

OSTEOCHONDROSES

Osteochondroses, also called aseptic necroses, are several diseases of children and adolescents characterized by death and regeneration of portion of bones without infection. These diseases are suspected clinically because of pain and tenderness of the involved area. The condition can be confirmed radiologically. There are several anatomic sites of involvement, depending on the affected bone. The two most significant osteochondroses are Legg-Perthes disease and Osgood-Schlatter disease. Legg-Perthes disease is an aseptic necrosis of the femoral head with onset during mid-childhood. Osgood-Schlatter disease is an aspetic necrosis of the anterior tibial tubercle seen in late childhood and early adolescence.

Orthopedic consultation is important in osteochondroses in order to prevent trauma of the involved bone and to allow proper regeneration.

SCOLIOSIS

Scoliosis is a lateral curvature of the spine. It may be idiopathic or may be caused by multiple conditions such as shortening of one leg, muscle spasms secondary to trauma, or structural defects of the spine.

Scoliosis that is not caused by muscle spasms secondary to an acute trauma always needs referral to an orthopedic surgeon in order to prevent or decrease future progression of the deformity.

Chapter 19
THE SKIN

The skin is one of the body systems and as such serves important physical, biochemical, physiologic, and psychologic functions. It is affected by numerous disease processes, including erythema toxicum, subcutaneous fat necrosis, diaper rash, impetigo, eczema, seborrheic dermatitis, tinea, pityriasis rosea, urticaria, papular urticaria, hemangiomas, and acne.

SOME NEONATAL SKIN DISORDERS

Certain common skin disorders occur only in the newborn. They are self-limited and require no treatment. However, the pediatric nurse practitioner needs to learn how to identify them to be able to reassure the mothers of infants with these problems. *Milia* are punctated, white, raised papules over the face and nose caused by retention of sebaceous material. *Mongolian spots* are bluish spots, often seen in the lower back, in babies of dark races. They are caused by a lack of even distribution of the normal skin pigment, melanin. *Subcutaneous fat necrosis* is seen as small hard nodules, usually on the back, cheeks, and buttocks and are probably due to birth trauma. The nurse practitioner needs to recognize *molding* of the neonatal head, which is a transiently misshaped head caused by pressure on the infant's skull by the mother's pelvic bones. This condition is not to be confused with cephalohematoma and caput succedaneum. *Cephalohematoma* is a collection of blood between the periosteum and the skull, which presents as a bulging fluid-filled mass confined to one bone of the skull. *Caput succedaneum* refers to swelling of the scalp due to birth trauma. Caput succedaneum crosses suture lines because the swelling is not confined to one bone of the skull. *Erythema toxicum* is a vesicular pustular rash on an erythematous base, which appears in newborns in the first 2 to 3 days of life and disappears in a few days. Examination under a microscope of scrapings from one of the lesions confirms the diagnosis by revealing numerous eosinophils.

DIAPER RASH

Diaper rash, or ammoniacal dermatitis, is an erythematous, vesicular, ulcerated eruption that occurs in the diaper area. It is generally caused by ammonia, which is produced by the action of the urea-splitting bacteria of the stool on the urea of the urine. Therefore, the main principle in treatment is to prevent contact of the skin with urea, which can be accomplished by decreasing the number of urea-splitting bacteria on the skin and by decreasing the contact of the urine with the skin. The former is done by washing the diaper area with soap and water every time the child has a bowel movement. Contact with urine is decreased by frequent diaper changes and by discouraging the constant use of rubber pants in order to allow for evaporation of the urine. In severe cases the child should be temporarily without· diapers. Diaper rash ointments decrease contact of the ammonia with the skin mechanically. They are also bactericidal and enhance skin healing.

When the skin is in good condition, the routine use of soap and water every time the child moves his bowels is all that is necessary to prevent diaper rash.

IMPETIGO

Impetigo is an infection of the skin. It is usually caused by group A beta hemolytic *Streptococcus* or by *Staphylococcus aureus* or by both.

The lesions may look vesicular, pustular, or bullous. Pustulovesicular lesions are the most common in impetigo. Bullous lesions are large vesicles that occur more often in newborn or younger infants, especially if the lesions are caused by *Staphylococcus aureus*. Since group A beta hemolytic *Streptococcus* often causes impetigo, complications such as nephritis may result.

Impetigo can be treated with local hygienic measures and topical antibiotics. However, treatment with systemic antibiotics such as penicillin is much more effective in preventing complications.

ECZEMA

Eczema is a common dermatitis in infancy and childhood. It usually appears before the age of 2 to 3 months and, although in a few cases eczema persists throughout life, it usually clears spontaneously by the time the child is 3 years old.

Numerous causes such as food allergens, environmental irritants and genetic predisposition are associated with eczema; however, the significance of each of these factors varies from person to person and in most cases the etiology of eczema remains unknown.

Clinically, the skin lesions are characterized by superficial inflammation, erythema, vesicles, and edema, which may look almost like burned skin. Since the lesions are very pruritic and the child scratches, infection often follows. Eventually, if the eczema continues to recur, thickening and lichenification of the involved skin occur. The initial lesions are usually on the cheeks, forehead, scalp, and flexure of the extremities. However, the entire skin may become involved.

In the management of eczema, infection always needs to be treated with systemic antibiotics. When the skin is not infected, it should be kept in good condition by anti-inflammatory measures, such as elimination of contact of wool against the skin, administration of anti-inflammatory drugs (topical steroid ointments), and humidifying ointments and hydrophilic bath oils that moisten the skin. Systemic antihistaminics are also helpful because of their antipruritic effect.

The value of an allergic evaluation, which consists mostly of an allergic history and elimination diet, is debatable but useful according to many. An elimination diet consists of restricting the diet to a simple nonallergenic diet for 10 days and then adding appropriate foods every 3 days to determine the possible causal relationship of any of these foods with exacerbation of the eczema. Elimination of the foods found to exacerbate the eczema is, of course, indicated. Skin tests in patients with eczema are almost useless.

SEBORRHEIC DERMATITIS

Seborrheic dermatitis is a common skin disease of early infancy. When it occurs in the scalp it is called cradle cap. In the older children seborrheic dermatitis produces dandruff.

In infancy seborrheic dermatitis resembles eczema, but it is usually more oily and less wet and also involves the skin behind the ears, axillae, and groin more frequently than does eczema.

Cradle cap usually requires no more treatment than vigorous washing and scrubbing of the scalp. There are numerous antidandruff shampoos available for the older child, which contain salicylic acid and sulfur. If the rest of the body is mildly involved, an antiseborrheic preparation containing sulfur, salicylic acid, and coal tar is used. If the involvement is severe, topical steroid preparations are of value.

URTICARIA

Urticaria, or hives, is an acute or chronically recurrent inflammation of the skin characterized by erythematous, sharply demarcated, red elevated patches, which are very pruritic.

There are many causes of hives. Food allergy, drug allergy, physical agents (such as heat), infections (such as some viral exanthems), and psychogenic factors are associated with urticaria; however, in most cases the cause remains unknown.

Both the itching and the lesions often respond to antihistaminic antipruritic medication such as diphenhydramine hydrochloride.

PAPULAR URTICARIA

Papular urticaria is characterized by pruritic papules followed by excoriation due to scratching.

Numerous etiologic theories have been postulated but most commonly the lesions seem to be caused by insects or parasites such as dog or cat fleas, bed bugs, mites, or lice.

Treatment consists of elimination of the cause and administration of antipruritic medications such as diphenhydramine to relieve itching.

TINEA

Tinea, or ringworm, infections are caused by fungi called epidermophytes, (fungi that stay on the epidermis). The numerous epidermophytes that attack man can be divided into *Microsporum* and *Trichophyton*. The former usually fluoresce under the Wood's light while the latter in general do not fluoresce.

Tinea infections are named according to the region of the body involved regardless of the specific organism causing the infection. For example, tinea capitis is a tinea infection of the scalp, and is often caused by *Microsporum auduini*. Tinea pedis, or athlete's foot, is a tinea infection of the feet, often caused by *Trichophyton rubrum*.

When mild, tinea infections are usually treated topically with Whitfield's ointment or some other topical antifungal agent. If they fail to respond to topical preparations they need to be treated systemically with oral griseofulvin, an antifungal agent.

PITYRIASIS ROSEA

Pityriasis rosea is a dermatologic disease of older children characterized by a pruritic papulosquamous eruption of acute onset. The cause is unknown but is thought to be viral.

Pityriasis rosea may be confused with tinea corporis, but in pityriasis rosea, characteristically, there is a herald patch or one large lesion that antecedes the others by 5 to 10 days. It is followed by a generalized spread of scaly erythematous pruritic patches, which tend to be parallel to the cleavage lines of the skin.

Pityriasis is a self-limiting disease but usually lasts 2 to 8 weeks. Only antipruritic medications are required.

HEMANGIOMAS

Hemangiomas are abnormal masses of blood vessels, which can be grouped into (1) flat capillary ("stork bite" or "port wine stain"), (2) raised capillary ("strawberry mark"), and (3) cavernous.

Flat capillary hemangiomas of small size ("stork bite") are commonly occurring pink spots often seen on the back of the neck, upper lip, and upper lids of newborns. No treatment is necessary since they usually disappear eventually. Large flat capillary hemangiomas ("port wine stain") are different. They are rare but do not disappear spontaneously and are frequently associated with convulsions and other neurologic disturbances.

Raised capillary hemangiomas ("strawberry marks") are slightly raised and sharply demarcated, bright red spots 2 to 3 cm in diameter. They frequently require no treatment and usually disappear by puberty.

Cavernous hemangiomas are bluish purple raised masses of blood vessels. Some will persist and may progress to large arteriovenous fistulae; however, most will grow until the child is 10 to 15 months of age and then will start to involute incompletely and therefore require surgery.

ACNE

Acne is caused by overactivity and plugging of the sebaceous glands. It commonly occurs during adolescence and young adulthood. The specific etiology is not known, although acne is probably related to hormonal changes during adolescence. Excessive caloric intake, especially of certain foods such as chocolate, nuts, and fatty and spicy foods, might exacerbate acne.

The treatment includes dietary management to avoid fatty foods, chocolate, and nuts; hygienic measurements such as local cleansing with soap and water; and in some cases keratolytic ointments. Opinions are divided regarding the value of dietary treatment. In severe cases the use of tetracycline orally is also beneficial.

Chapter 20

THE NERVOUS SYSTEM

The evaluation of the nervous system is one of the most difficult parts of the physical examination. The neurologist views the nervous system as an electrical system that can be evaluated by physical examination, whereas the psychiatrist or psychologist views its functioning in human interaction.

In the practice of pediatrics, conditions such as meningitis, epilepsy, hyperactivity, cerebral palsy, and mental retardation are neurologic diseases of common occurrence and will be considered in this chapter. Fever, although not a neurologic problem per se is also discussed in this chapter because of its close relationship with febrile convulsions. Psychiatric problems and problems of human interaction will be discussed in Chapter 21.

MENINGITIS

Meningitis is an infection of the meninges, or membranes, which cover the brain and spinal cord. Unless a high index of suspicion is entertained it is often missed; it should therefore be suspected clinically when an infant has a febrile illness with paradoxical irritability. The older child usually has fever and malaise in addition to the more classic symptoms of meningeal irritation, such as headache and projectile vomiting.

The physical examination characteristically reveals a child in varying states of consciousness (from alertness to coma) with signs of meningeal irritation such as stiff neck and Kernig and Brudzinski signs. These symptoms are more commonly present in older children than in infants (see Chapter 3).

Examination of the spinal fluid, which must include cultures, is conclusive in arriving at a correct diagnosis (see Chapter 7). Before a definite etiologic diagnosis is made, ampicillin is usually given in doses of 300 to 400 mg per kilogram of body weight, intravenously. In the newborn antibiotics such as kanamycin are used, since microorganisms unaffected by ampicillin, such as coliform bacilli, are frequently involved.

FEVER

Fever, an increase in temperature above normal, is a common reason for parents to seek medical care for their children. Fever itself is usually not dangerous and the parents need reassurance. The underlying cause of the fever is what requires treatment. Febrile convulsions will be discussed later in this

104

chapter. Antipyretic agents, such as aspirin or acetoaminophen, and sponging the child with tepid water are effective in decreasing the temperature.

CONVULSIONS

Convulsions are common in children and the diagnosis differs according to age groups—newborn period, early childhood, and late childhood.

In the *newborn* infant the most common conditions responsible for convulsions are anoxia and hemorrhage secondary to birth trauma; metabolic problems (such as hypocalcemia, which produces tetany of the newborn, and hypoglycemia in infants of diabetic mothers and in those small for their gestational age); and congenital illnesses or anomalies of the central nervous system. In *early childhood* conditions such as intracranial infection (meningitis) and extracranial infection (fever) are the most likely causes of convulsions. In *older children* epilepsy or idiopathic convulsive disorders and tumors predominate as causative agents for convulsions.

Febrile convulsions. Febrile convulsions are common, occurring in approximately 10 percent of all children. As the name suggests, febrile convulsions are convulsions associated with fever from any cause; they are benign and eventually disappear. However, since the first convulsion of idiopathic epilepsy often occurs with fever, clinicians need certain criteria to determine whether the convulsions are simple febrile convulsions or are the beginning of idiopathic epilepsy. Febrile convulsions should comply with the following criteria: they have to occur in neurologically normal children; they have to be generalized and to last less than 10 minutes; they have to occur during the first 18 hours of a particular febrile episode; the age of onset has to be between 6 months and 4 years; they should leave no residual neurologic abnormalities; and the electroencephalograms, if obtained, should be normal after 2 weeks.

A young infant with the first febrile convulsion usually requires a spinal tap to exclude the possibility of meningitis. This is rarely required in older children with subsequent febrile convulsions. Opinions vary regarding the use of anticonvulsant drugs after a febrile seizure. Most physicians use phenobarbital during the remainder of the febrile illness while some believe the patient should receive the drug for 1 year following the seizure.

BREATH-HOLDING SPELLS

Breath-holding spells are not seizures; they occur in response to frustration in a similar fashion to temper tantrums in children with a poor mother-child relationship or other stressful environmental factors.

Classically, the child cries, breathes deeply a few times and then holds his breath until he turns blue, becomes rigid, and falls on the floor unconscious. As soon as he loses consciousness he starts breathing. Since breath-holding spells are not seizures, these children will have a normal electroencephalogram. These spells are benign; that is, they do not cause brain damage.

Therapy should be geared to improve the mother-child relationship. The child, however, should not get special attention during the spells because this is what he is looking for, and if he obtains it he will continue to have spells.

HYPERACTIVITY

Hyperactivity, "minimal brain damage," and "hyperkinetic syndrome" are terms used somewhat interchangeably for a diagnosis which is being made with increasing frequency. This diagnosis implies that there is brain damage and some educators are especially prone to the idea that hyperactive children are damaged children. However, there is no proof of brain damage in hyperactive children, and there are probably many causes of the syndrome.

Some of these hyperactive children have either intellectual limitations or, more commonly, visual-motor limitations that are unrecognized by their parents or teachers. These children cannot cope with problem-solving situations appropriate to their age group, and therefore are frustrated and react with hyperactivity. Other hyperactive children are frustrated psychologically because of the interpersonal relations at home. Finally, many hyperactive children have a combination of both organic dysfunctions and psychologic problems.

The first group, in which there is frustration on an objective basis, needs to be treated by decreasing the environmental expectations—the expectations of the school and parents. The second group is best handled by correcting the underlying psychologic problems through family counseling. Counseling is most important for all hyperactive children, regardless of the cause.

Numerous drugs are commonly used in the treatment of hyperactive children. These drugs are either cataleptic drugs, such as dextroamphetamine or methylphenidate; tranquilizers, such as chlorpromazine; or sedatives, such as diphenhydramine. Cataleptics are particularly useful in those hyperactive children with visual-motor incoordination. Drug therapy can be useful but by no means should it be the sole means of therapy.

MENTAL RETARDATION

Mental retardation refers to a reduced rate of cognitive growth, whether in the attainment of knowledge or in the development of one or more cognitive abilities.

Mental retardation should be suspected during routine health appraisal if the developmental milestones are significantly delayed or if the child performs below his age group in one of the several developmental screening tests such as the Denver Developmental Scale (see Chapter 6). Although there are numerous causes of mental retardation, most often the cause is unknown. However, when mental retardation is suspected, a thorough diagnostic evaluation is always in order not only to elucidate the causes but also because other pathologic conditions such as congenital heart disease are frequently associated with this diagnosis.

The management of mental retardation is complex and usually involves a team effort, which includes physician, school nurse, social workers, and special education teachers. Social workers often coordinate the efforts of the other team members.

CEREBRAL PALSY

According to the United Cerebral Palsy Association, "cerebral palsy is a group of conditions, usually originating in childhood, characterized by paralysis, weakness, incoordination or any other alienation of motor function caused by pathology of the motor centers of the brain." It is frequently associated with convulsions, intellectual impairment, and specific learning disabilities. The causes of the injury to the brain include anoxia, infection, and birth trauma.

The pediatric nurse practitioner should realize that many children with gross motor abnormalities have greater intelligence than is immediately apparent. The accurate assessment of these children's intelligence is often difficult but necessary. Since the problems associated with cerebral palsy are many and varied, its management requires a team approach that includes a physician, social worker, physical therapist, and special education teachers. Each of these disciplines is of extreme importance in enabling a child with cerebral palsy to attain his maximal functional potential.

Chapter 21

PSYCHOLOGIC DISORDERS

Psychologic disorders in children, because of their frequency and significance, are an important part of pediatric practice. Any health worker involved with children needs to be familiar with these problems in order to handle children with psychologic problems more effectively.

Some psychologic diseases and other psychologic topics have been covered elsewhere in this book (psychosexual development, Chapter 6; encopresis, Chapter 15; enuresis, Chapter 16; hyperactivity, Chapter 20; parental substitution and child abuse, Chapter 25; school problems, Chapter 26; and some emotional problems of the adolescent, Chapter 27). In this chapter the nurse practitioner will become familiar with a classification of mental illnesses and with some specific details of the most frequently encountered developmental and situational problems.

In order of increasing severity, psychologic disorders of children can be classified as developmental disorders, situational disorders, neurotic disorders, character disorders, and psychotic disorders. A separate category groups the psychologic disorders associated with organic brain damage, although the interrelationship between organic brain damage and behavior is often difficult to explain, as exemplified in the hyperactive child syndrome (see Chapter 20).

DEVELOPMENTAL DISORDERS

Developmental disorders are expected problems associated with successive stages of psychosexual development.

These disorders are numerous and a few examples are: excessive crying during the neonatal period, feeding problems during infancy, tantrum and night terrors during the toddler years, phobias during the preschool years, excessive shyness or extreme acting out during school years, and acting out during adolescence.

In general no treatment is needed for these developmental disorders. If the symptoms increase to become severe, counseling should be attempted to make the parents understand that these disorders are most likely not fixed and that they will disappear with time and proper management.

SITUATIONAL DISORDERS

Situational, or reactive, disorders arise from environmental situations that are abnormal for a given child at a given age and with which he is unable to cope. In situational disorders the problem is usually caused by faulty or inappropriate parental attitudes. These attitudes are easily apparent and can be perceived and identified as such by the child. For example, open parental rejection or overanxiety may be the faulty attitude behind many situational disorders.

Examples of situational disorders are: thumbsucking after 5 years of age, obesity, nail biting, breath-holding spells, teeth grinding, pica, head banging, excessive masturbation, and enuresis (see Chapters 15 and 16).

Treatment in younger children attempts to decrease the unhealthy interaction between the child and his parents. In older children and adolescents most of the therapeutic effort is done with the child himself; in fact, a clear-cut alliance with the adolescent and not with the parents is extremely important in therapy.

NEUROSES, CHARACTER DISORDERS, AND PSYCHOSES

Neurotic disorders are manifested by a high degree of anxiety. Their development seems to start with a masked faulty parental attitude of which the child is not usually aware. For example, open and clear parental rejection often leads to a situational disorder in the child; masked parental rejection gradually leads to the child's internalization of the conflict. The child represses the conflict into his subconscious, a process which causes the high anxiety of neurotic disorders.

Internalization is also essential to character disorders, but in these cases the child's early relationships with other people have had a more adverse effect on his equilibrium and, therefore, he is more unstable. He develops lack of awareness of anxiety and lack of insight as defense mechanisms.

Since the process of internalization is essential to both neurotic and character disorders, these problems are first seen in older children and adolescents. An example of neurotic and character disorders can be found in a child with a learning problem. A child with a neurotic learning problem is very anxious and, although he knows his anxiety is useless, he fails to recognize that the anxiety is due to an internal conflict. Furthermore, he is unable to stop the anxiety in spite of the fact that he recognizes the consequences of his learning problem. On the other hand, a child with a learning problem due to a character disorder has no anxiety. He knows that he is having learning problems, but he is unable to see the future consequences of his lack of learning.

In more severe problems such as psychotic problems contact with reality is permanently or transitorily lost; an example of a psychotic problem is infantile autism in which the child does not relate to people at all.

All children with these problems—neuroses, character disorders, and psychoses—need to be referred to a child guidance clinic or other psychiatric facility. Psychiatric hospitals, unfortunately, are usually overcrowded and, therefore, it is best to refer the family to a child guidance clinic or a pediatric clinic with guidance facilities. The clinic, in turn, either handles the problem or refers the family to a psychiatric hospital.

SOME COMMON PROBLEMS

Toilet training. Bladder and bowel training are important for healthy psychologic development. Most children are not ready for bowel training until age 2 to 3 years and for bladder training until a few months later. Any attempt to train the child before he is ready can only be detrimental to the mother-child relationship. The use of bowel softeners, suppositories, and enemas is also undesirable. When the child is ready, which is usually when he can communicate his needs, the parents need to let him try and to praise him if he is successful.

Thumbsucking. Thumbsucking is often a sign of insecurity or, according to some authors, a sign of insufficient sucking activity during infancy. It tends to disappear in many children before the end of the first year and in most before 6 years of age.

Thumbsucking in infancy needs no treatment, short of possibly increasing sucking time, either by using a smaller hole in the nipple for artificially fed infants or prolonging nursing time in breast-fed infants.

In handling thumbsucking in older children the nurse practitioner needs to evaluate the total family situation and should help the family in facing the basis of the child's insecurity. In older children the promise of a reward and the application of a reminder, such as a bitter substance to the thumb, may help.

Sleep disturbances. Separation anxiety at the end of the first year and fear of loss of control over aggression later in childhood often cause sleep disturbances.

The nurse practitioner needs to evaluate the interpersonal relationships at home. Parents often need advice so they can reassure the child either verbally or at times physically (by going to the child's room) when the child wakes up at night. At the same time the parents should be warned against bringing the child to their bed because this may produce more tension in the child (see Oedipal complex in Chapter 6).

Negativism. All children go through a period called psychologic negativism during the ages of approximately 18 months to 2½ years. However, persistence of this normal negativism into the preschool years (between the ages of 3 and 6 years) is commonly a manifestation of emotional problems.

The nurse practitioner will usually find a tense, withdrawn child who tends to refuse everything and who lies frequently. The parents of such children are often overauthoritative, overcritical, and overcorrective.

Negativistic children between the ages of 3 and 6 years are best handled in a group such as a nursery school or kindergarten where the teacher can invite, but not force, the child to participate in group activities. The parents need counseling regarding the child's need for praise and acceptance.

Speech defects. The major speech defects are stuttering (repetition of certain syllables), stammering (blocking during speech), articulation defects, immature or babyish speech, and delayed speech.

Stuttering and stammering occur transiently in many children, especially in boys between the ages of 2 and 4 years. Adequate counseling of the parents is of utmost importance, because persistent stuttering may result if too much attention is paid to the child's difficulty. Parents should be reassured that stuttering during this age is a developmental pattern that will disappear spontaneously provided the parents listen attentively and patiently to the child, do not attempt to correct him or to finish a word for him, and do not ask the child to "start over again and say it slowly." If parents are unable to follow this advice or if the stuttering does not improve significantly within a year, further evaluation by a speech therapist or a psychologist is usually indicated. A school-age child who stutters is a difficult problem beyond the capabilities of the pediatric nurse practitioner and deserves further evaluation by a speech therapist and often by a psychologist.

Mild articulation defects, such as omission or substitution of consonants are common during the preschool years. The vast majority of these defects will be corrected spontaneously by age 7. However, the response to treatment by a speech therapist is usually very prompt and may be recommended at 4½ years of age to save the child embarrassment and teasing when he starts school. Immature, babyish speech also usually responds well to simple management. The parents should not treat the child as a baby and should not talk to him in baby talk.

Delayed speech may be associated with immature speech, but it may also be a sign of mental retardation or hearing impairment; thus, children with significantly delayed speech should be evaluated by a competent audiologist and psychologist.

Temper tantrums. Temper tantrums due to frustration occur frequently at the end of the second year of life. The nurse practitioner needs to talk with the family to elucidate and attempt to correct the sources of frustration (see also Breath-holding spells in Chapter 20). It is essential to improve the child's interpersonal relationships and to ignore or to handle the child in a matter-of-fact way when he is having his temper tantrum; attention at the time of the episode will only reinforce this pattern of behavior. The parent should either ignore the tantrum or put the child in his room with the admonition that he is welcome to come out when he feels he can behave.

Masturbation. Parents and children have often heard numerous opinions regarding masturbation, ranging from a very rigid authoritarian approach to a very permissive approach.

Masturbation in infants and young children is not uncommon and often indicates lack of social stimulation (boredom). In older children and adolescents masturbation relates to exploration, experimentation, and gratification of the newly developed sexual instinct.

Parents of infants and young children need reassurance that masturbation is not physically dangerous. The child needs examination to eliminate possible causes of irritation such as pinworm infestation, and the habit should be discouraged by pointing out that this is an infantile habit like thumb-sucking. More importantly, however, parents should offer positive alternatives.

In adolescents, masturbation can only be handled through a value system and intellectual understanding, but the adolescent needs reassurance that the habit is not physically dangerous.

Rhythmic motor habits. Rhythmic movements such as head rolling, head banging, and body or bed rocking are not uncommon in infants and children.

In head rolling the infant moves the head rhythmically so vigorously that he often rubs off the hair from the back of the head. In head nodding the infant either rhythmically nods or shakes the head laterally, and in body rocking he usually sits or semi-kneels and moves the body rhythmically.

Theories regarding the psychopathology of rhythmic body habits are numerous, but emotional deprivation is high on the list of possibilities. Thus the nurse practitioner needs to evaluate the family to determine the conditions producing the lack of social stimulation.

Nail biting. Nail biting is usually a sign of tension which is manifested in children at approximately 4 years of age. In these cases the nurse practitioner needs to investigate and try to relieve the situation producing tension for the child.

Tics. Tics or habit spasms are recurrent, abrupt, purposeless, involuntary movements of circumscribed muscle groups. They often are a clinical problem between ages 8 and 12 years and usually indicate tension at home.

Most tics are mild and require no treatment. In severe tics the nurse practitioner needs to try to correct any possible source of irritation and to make an effort to correct the conflict producing situation. However, referral is often necessary since severe tics are difficult to manage.

Acting out. Acting out is usually an expression of aggressive or sexual instincts or both; most commonly it becomes antisocial or delinquent. Psychopathologically, acting out is associated with numerous factors, such as lack of early attachment to people (as in the case of foster children who are sent from one home to another) or with fulfilling the unconscious wishes of the parents (as in the case of a delinquent who, by his behavior, is really doing what his father subconsciously would like to have done).

In most instances the child needs firmness and protection from his impulses as well as proper attention to his psychologic needs to be able to change the behavior before legal authorities become involved. Once legal authorities become involved the health professional must make legal authorities aware of the health problems of the patient.

Chapter 22

PHARMACOLOGY

The purpose of this chapter is to familiarize the pediatric nurse practitioner with some basic drugs used in the management of pediatric patients on an ambulatory basis. The intention of this chapter is not to enable pediatric nurse practitioners to prescribe drugs but to make them more educated members of the health team. They will then be able to determine the significance of accidental overdosage as well as the most likely therapy for certain illnesses in order to alert physicians about possible errors in medications.

ROUTE

As is well known to nurses, the principal routes of administration are oral, rectal, intramuscular, intravenous, subcutaneous, and topical.

The oral route, which in many drugs produces very acceptable therapeutic blood levels, is the most commonly used route in ambulatory pediatrics because of the ease of administration. This route, of course, should not be used for children with nausea and vomiting.

DOSAGE

In pediatrics most drug dosages are calculated either on the basis of weight or on the basis of surface area. Available charts called nomograms help in determining surface area after the body weight and height are known. It is important to remember that children are not small adults, particularly during the neonatal period when the child is not only small but the level of maturation of the organ systems is different not only from adults but from older children as well. Therefore, extrapolation from adult dosages on a weight basis is not always appropriate; for example, the newborn liver and kidney do not have the same capacity per unit as the adult organs and drugs excreted through these organs will accumulate rapidly in the bodies of newborns. However, there are rules to convert adult doses into children's doses, which can be used only as rough guides and only with drugs that do not require extremely exact dosage. One of these rules is the rule of Clark in which the adult dose is multiplied by the child's weight divided by 150.

$$\text{Child's dose} = \text{adult dose} \times \frac{\text{child's weight}}{150}$$

ADVERSE REACTIONS

Adverse reactions to drugs are due to overdose, side effects, allergy, idiosyncrasy, and developmental problems.

Overdose, as the name implies, is an expected undesirable effect of a drug because of the large dose administered (for example, cardiac arrhythmia due to a large dose of digitalis).

Side effects are undesirable effects of a drug which can and will happen with predictable frequency in the usual dose of a drug (for example, diarrhea is a common side effect after administration of ampicillin).

Allergic reaction is an undesirable effect due to antibodies produced by the host against a particular drug (for example, anaphylaxis with penicillin).

Idiosyncrasy is also an undesirable effect of a drug which is unpredictable and for which there is no explanation (as photosensitivity rash upon exposure to light in a few individuals taking sulfonamide).

Developmental adverse reactions are reactions that occur with certain drugs and are directly related to the level of developmental maturation of the patient (for example, malformations in the unborn child due to thalidomide or staining of developing teeth by tetracyclines).

DRUGS IN AMBULATORY PEDIATRICS

The pediatric nurse practitioner needs familiarity with certain drugs that are frequently used in the practice of pediatrics. For didactic purposes these drugs will be grouped according to function.

Analgesics. Analgesics are drugs that diminish pain and are either *narcotic* or *nonnarcotic.* Drugs in the *narcotic* group, such as codeine and morphine, may produce addiction (see Chapter 27) if administered repeatedly. *Nonnarcotic* analgesics are not as effective in diminishing pain as the narcotics but they do not produce addiction. Some nonnarcotic analgesics are also widely utilized for their antipyretic effect, such as acetylsalicylic acid (aspirin), salicylamide (Liquiprim), and acetominophen (Tempra, Tylenol).

Anthelmintics. Anthelmintics are drugs used in the treatment of parasites. Since in the United States today the most significant parasite is *Enterobius vermicularis* (pinworm), the nurse practitioner needs to know that pyrvinium pamoate (Povan) is at present the most effective and safest drug to eradicate pinworm infestation. The drug stains the stool red, and the patient or his parents should be told of this side effect.

Antibacterials. Drugs that are bacteriostatic (prevent bacterial multiplication) and bactericidal (kill bacteria) are essential in pediatrics since bacterial infections account for many illnesses in children. Most of these drugs are antibiotics such as penicillin and erythromycin, but a few are synthetic chemicals such as sulfonamide.

Penicillins are divided into penicillin G, which is the oldest one; penicillin V, which is acid resistant; and semisynthetic penicillins, which are further subdivided into those which are penicillinase resistant, such as methicillin and oxacillin, and those which are broad in spectrum, such as ampicillin. Penicillins are extremely safe drugs; the major adverse reactions are allergic reactions which range from simple urticaria to severe anaphylaxis.

Penicillin G is a very effective bactericidal agent against many gram positive organisms (see Chapter 7) such as streptococci and pneumococci. Benzathine penicillin G has the same spectrum as penicillin G but it stays in the body longer. Combinations of penicillin G together with benzathine penicillin G produce a rapid blood level due to the penicillin G, followed by a slower rising blood level which persists due to the benzathine penicillin G. Benzathine penicillin G alone produces a low blood level that lasts for a month and thus is utilized in the prophylactic care of patients after rheumatic fever.

Penicillin V has an antimicrobial spectrum similar to that of penicillin G but is resistant to the acid of the stomach and is therefore better absorbed when administered orally.

Penicillinase-resistant penicillins such as methicillin and oxacillin are useful in treating patients with staphylococcal infection caused by organisms which produce penicillinase, an enzyme that destroys other penicillins.

Broad-spectrum penicillins such as ampicillin are bactericidal not only against gram-positive but also against many gram-negative organisms such as *Hemophilus influenzae;* however, broad-spectrum antibiotics frequently produce diarrhea.

Erythromycin is similar in antibacterial spectrum to penicillin G except for a slightly broader spectrum against some gram-negative organisms such as *Hemophilus influenzae.* The main usefulness of erythromycin is as a substitute for penicillin in patients allergic to penicillin and in the treatment of a few specific infections such as pertussis and mycoplasma pneumonia.

Sulfonamides are not antibiotics but are inexpensive synthetic chemicals; however, they are good antibacterial agents. In pediatrics sulfonamides are primarily used in urinary tract infection and occasionally in other specific infections such as *Hemophilus influenzae* laryngotracheobronchitis.

Antifungals. There are two commonly utilized antifungal agents in ambulatory pediatrics: griseofulvin for epidermophytic skin infection (such as ringworm) and mycostatin for *Candida albicans* (monilia) infection (such as thrush).

Antivirals. At present most antiviral agents are not very effective and are usually very toxic. 5-Iodouridine is used topically in cases of herpes simplex of the eye.

Anticonvulsants. There are many anticonvulsants and some of the most important are phenobarbital, diphenylhydantoin (Dilantin), diazepam (Valium), paraldehyde, and trimethadione.

Phenobarbital is very inexpensive and very safe. It is one of the most commonly used agents to stop as well as to prevent convulsions. *Diazepam* (Valium) is also used frequently to stop seizures. *Paraldehyde* has the advantage of being excreted through the respiratory tract and therefore the status of the patient's kidney and liver is unimportant.

Dilantin alone or together with phenobarbital is commonly used in patients with grand mal convulsions. *Trimethadione* is a major drug against petit mal convulsions.

Antihistaminics. Antihistaminics are essential for the management of the allergic patient. Some common ones are *diphenhydramine hydrochloride* (Benadryl) and *chlorpheniramine* (Chlortrimeton).

Combinations of an antihistaminic with an adrenergic vasoconstrictor compound are commonly used as decongestants, for example, actidyl-pseudo-ephedrine (Actifed).

Bronchodilators. Bronchodilators are essential in the management of asthmatic patients, since they counteract the major problems in asthma— bronchospasm and hypersecretion. Some examples are *epinephrine* (Adrenalin, Sus-Phrine), *aminophylline,* and combinations of bronchodilators such as *theophylline-ephedrine* combined with phenobarbital (Tedral).

Emetics. Emetics, or drugs to induce vomiting, are important in the treatment of poisoning. The major emetics are apomorphine and ipecac. *Apomorphine* may produce respiratory depression and is a narcotic; thus, it is not frequently utilized. Syrup of *ipecac* is an effective emetic which, when given appropriately, is so safe that it has been recommended for home use before the child is brought to a medical facility. However, if given in extremely large doses, it may produce cardiotoxicity (see Chapter 11).

Hematinics. Hematinics are drugs utilized in anemia to improve the condition of the blood. As mentioned in Chapter 9 iron deficiency is a common pediatric problem for which iron salts such as ferrous sulfates are curative.

Psychoactives. Psychoactive drugs are numerous and the illicit utilization of these drugs among adolescents is increasing at an incredible speed (see Chapter 27).

In children psychoactive drugs are used therapeutically in several disease states such as hyperactive child syndrome (see Chapter 20) for which both *dextroamphetamine* (Dexedrine) and *methylphenidate hydrochloride* (Ritalin) are used. If neither one of these drugs is useful, antihistaminics (such as diphenhydramine) which produce sedation, or tranquilizers may be required.

SECTION III

SOCIAL PROBLEMS

Chapter 23

HEALTH CARE DELIVERY

During the first 50 years of this century teaching and research in medical schools were primarily concerned with the biologic basis of disease. Investigation in the basic sciences—microbiology, biochemistry, and physiology— was greatly emphasized, and gradually clinical medicine became organ system- and disease-oriented rather than a comprehensive program concerned with the patient as a total person and a member of a community.

More recently a generalized reevaluation of goals and priorities in society has brought renewed interaction between medical schools and communities. Medical schools are becoming increasingly aware of the fact that they are responsible not only for the adequate transmission of medical knowledge but also for the fostering of correct attitudes of commitment and service through delivery of comprehensive medical care to the community. Community action through service and health care research have become integral parts of the programs of numerous medical schools in this country.

Accomplishment of broad goals of expanded medical care have been hampered by a severe shortage of both physicians and other trained medical personnel. To cope with the shortage of manpower in pediatrics, programs to train nurses as pediatric nurse practitioners and programs to train other paramedical health workers have been developed.

The present chapter will briefly discuss pediatrics as traditionally practiced. It will also consider the scope of different community resources that can be of value in the present and future practice of pediatrics.

MEDICAL PRACTICE

Until World War II, medical practice in the United States had been on a fee-for-service basis in which individual physicians were in private practice. Since World War II there has been a definite trend, first, toward group practice, then gradually toward prepaid group practice. More recently, the trend has been toward the development of neighborhood health centers.

The pattern that is clearly emerging in medical practice in the United States shows two types of facilities: (1) those facilities caring for patients on a continuous basis, the so-called *primary care* facilities, and (2) those giving special episodic care, the so-called *secondary care* facilities.

Primary care facilities provide treatment and health supervision to patients over long periods of time. Episodic, or secondary, care facilities are used only when the nature of the illness demands specialized care (for example, major surgery) or when the care is needed on an emergency basis.

Before World War II primary care was given principally by individual physicians on a fee-for-service basis. In this set-up a well-trained nurse, assistant, or associate was of the utmost importance, and for years physicians have been depending on this individually trained professional.

Since World War II there has been a definite trend toward group practice and, more recently, toward prepaid group practice. In a prepaid group practice the patient or his family pays a specific amount per month for which the group provides the family with medical care. Again, the role of a well-trained nurse is essential. More recently, neighborhood health centers have arisen in urban ghettos. Neighborhood clinics are small facilities delivering primary care to persons living in the immediate area. These centers are usually administered by a community board and are supported in part by the government, either through a grant or through the collection of fees from a government-sponsored program. In such clinics the role of the pediatric nurse practitioner is essential.

Secondary care facilities, located in hospitals, are those facilities to which the patient comes for episodic care. Secondary care centers provide long-term care for a small number of patients, but most patients are returned to the primary care centers for follow-up.

Pediatric nurse practitioner programs are geared to train nurses to practice in primary care facilities. However, pediatric nurse practitioners may also be useful in certain secondary care facilities such as the emergency room or a cystic fibrosis clinic.

COMMUNITY NURSING SERVICES

Community nursing facilities are an important arm of any ambulatory care center since they are often the only direct extension into the patient's home. Community nursing agencies perform both preventive and therapeutic services. Some are official agencies, such as the nursing division of the city or county health department; others are voluntary agencies, such as the Visiting Nurse Association. Others are not independent agencies but are home care branches of health programs of specific institutions.

Public health nurses from county or city health departments primarily perform preventive and health-promoting services through well-baby clinics and home visits to selected groups of mothers. In well-baby clinics the public health nurse not only administers immunizations but also attempts to give as complete a service of health education as possible. The public health nurse also visits selected groups of mothers (such as the mothers of premature infants and teen-age mothers) to educate these women in the essentials of health care.

The Visiting Nurse Association is a voluntary agency that brings nursing care into the home. Visiting nurses may not only provide health education but may also deliver some specific nursing care, such as caring for a burned or a chronically ill patient at home.

In addition to public health and visiting nurses, ambulatory pediatric care facilities are sometimes able to provide their patients with nursing services at home because they have their own team of nurses to deliver such a service. Although an independent team of nurses to provide health services at home is expensive, such a team greatly enlarges the scope of services of an ambulatory care facility.

Pediatric nurse practitioners need to investigate the specific facilities available in the community in order to utilize the services of community nursing agencies to their fullest extent.

HOMEMAKING SERVICES

Homemaking services are provided by several agencies. Their goal is to temporarily help a family in need by taking over some or most of the housekeeping chores. These agencies are nonprofit, and may be public or private.

Homemaker health aides are selected women who should be warm, mature, and experienced in rearing children. These women are given an intensive course of about 30 hours and are supervised in their work by public health nurses or social workers.

By utilizing the services of a homemaker aide, the pediatric nurse practitioner could greatly help a family through difficult periods, such as when the mother of the family becomes ill and is unable to perform her usual housekeeping chores.

COMMUNITY PSYCHOLOGIC SERVICES

The need for psychologic counseling services on an outpatient basis far exceeds the availability of such services. Thus pediatricians and pediatric clinics delivering primary pediatric care should become involved in such counseling. However, there are also community resources that offer psychologic diagnostic and therapeutic services for a selected number of children.

The most commonly utilized community resource offering psychologic services is the psychologic service office of the board of education or, in some cases, of the individual school. The school social worker in some schools delivers counseling services. Child guidance clinics and family service organizations are also essential in providing psychologic services to a community.

Prior to referral to a community agency the nurse practitioner needs to know the facilities available in that particular agency and the period of time expected to elapse before the patient is actually seen. The nurse practitioner must remember that there is nothing more frustrating to a patient than waiting several months for an appointment only to be finally informed that that institution does not handle his particular type of problem.

GOVERNMENT PROGRAMS

Government programs concerned with the physical and emotional health of children are numerous. They usually provide economic support and they usually dictate policies with which the recipient needs to comply in order to maintain the economic support. Most of these programs are supported from both federal and state sources; often they are initiated with federal money, but usually there is a compulsory state matching fund requirement.

At the federal government level, health and welfare programs are generally under the Department of Health, Education and Welfare and can be grouped into rehabilitation services, children's services, and medical services.

Government programs of rehabilitation services such as those for crippled children or the mentally retarded usually pay for services and set standards of care. For example, the Crippled Children's Commission pays for services rendered to children with chronic disabilities provided both the institution and the person rendering the service meet specific standards.

Children's Bureau programs are mostly concerned with maternal and child health, maternal and infant care, and child welfare programs. Children and youth grants are provided, which are geared to provide economic support in order to develop models of primary care facilities for children.

Medical services such as Medicare and Medicaid (Title XIX) programs pay for certain medical services for specific segments of the population. The Medicaid program pays for therapeutic medical services on a fee-for-service basis. Admission to the program is based on an economic scale, and patients can only seek services at the time of an illness. The program does not provide for health supervision of well patients.

The pediatric nurse practitioner should understand that the above-mentioned government programs are constantly changing and must therefore be aware of new developments in government involvement in the health field both at the federal and at the state level.

Chapter 24

THE EXPANDED ROLE OF
THE NURSE*

It has been said that the health of all the people is really the foundation upon which all their happiness and all their strengths as a community depend. The nursing profession has always been dedicated to the preservation and restoration of health. As medical science progressed and consequently expanded the role of the physician, nurses were in the forefront to fill in the gaps created. They willingly and effectively assumed health care functions previously considered to be the physician's. However, health care needs in this country are still far from being met. Changes in patterns of delivery will continue, and it is generally believed that greater emphasis will be on care outside the hospital in a wider variety of health care facilities. We are already seeing the development of neighborhood health clinics, and emphasis is being placed on prevention of disease. The critical shortages of health manpower, particularly physicians, has been discussed in previous chapters. We need to intensify our efforts to overcome inefficiencies in the use of all health personnel. Nursing has already taken a second look to ascertain its role in helping to relieve a critical situation. One area of need is that of a pediatric nurse practitioner. A crisis now exists in providing health care for a growing population of children. More and better care to children can be provided only through increased and more effective utilization of adequately trained allied health professionals, particularly nurses.

Studies pertaining to the growth of the concept of a pediatric nurse practitioner have been published since the mid-Sixties. Since the beginning both

*By Sister Mary Noreen McGowan, R.N., M.S., P.N.P., Associate Professor of Nursing, St. Louis University School of Nursing and Allied Health Professions; Lois Sullivan, R.N., M.S., Director of Nursing, Cardinal Glennon Memorial Hospital for Children; Dianne Cohen, R.N., B.S., P.N.P.; Janice Kocur, R.N., B.S., P.N.P.; Barbara Metzger, R.N., P.N.P.; Barbara Tournour, R.N., P.N.P.; Karen Worley, R.N., P.N.P. Edited by Rita Lavedier, R.N., M.S., Associate Professor and Director of Undergraduate Education, St. Louis University School of Nursing and Allied Health Professions.

the concept of this new role for the pediatric nurse and the programs of retraining have been highly controversial. Differences of opinion focus on type and length of training considered necessary to prepare the nurse for this role. Nurse educators do have consensus on one issue—that continued education is necessary. Basic nursing education prepares the nurse in health maintenance skills and to care for ill children. The nurse has also learned the process of scientific problem-solving leading to sound judgment and decision-making. The nurse knows how to assess patient needs. Physical assessment using traditional medical techniques is a relatively minor extension of conventional nursing assessment. The value of a pediatric assistant program is that the nurse not only learns some new skills but also is given practice in those previously learned.

It is generally agreed that nurses are well prepared and able to assume responsibility for primary, family-oriented child care and child health supervision in a variety of settings. Thus, in order to extend the role to performing specific medical care functions, the nurse needs a relatively short period of continued education to attain the proficiency and competency needed to perform the new technical skills associated with the expanded role. Any pediatric assistant program should be built on previously mastered nursing knowledge and skills. Additional emphasis is given to the areas of normal growth and development, patient assessment, interviewing and counseling, family teaching, childhood illnesses, and child health care services.

The pediatric nurse practitioner can strengthen the nursing role in public health clinics, pediatrician's private practice offices, out-patient clinics, neighborhood health clinics, and community projects for children. The nurse's knowledge and skills could well be put to use in emergency rooms of childrens' hospitals. However, the nurse practitioner's specific role is difficult to define because there are so many variables to consider in the types of settings in which he or she can function.

It seems, then, that the pediatric nurse practitioner can make a valuable contribution toward alleviating human needs and the manpower shortage. The need is urgent and nurses are already demonstrating that they can improve the quality of pediatric care.

The American Academy of Pediatrics has adopted the official position that "a physician may delegate the responsibility of providing appropriate portions of health examinations and health care for infants to a properly trained individual working under his supervision." The academy suggested three levels. They are:

1. Pediatric nurse associate: A registered nurse who has completed a recognized training program, usually a 16-week course.
2. Pediatric office assistant: A practical nurse who has completed a recog-

nized program longer than that required for the registered nurse, or any person with 2 years of college who has completed such a program.

3. Pediatric aide: A person with a high school diploma or the equivalent who is trained on the job by a board-certified pediatrician.

The American Nurses' Association and the American Academy of Pediatrics have collaborated and issued joint statements concerning the changes taking place in health care services to children. Guidelines and concepts for short-term continuing education courses were developed and published in the *American Journal of Nursing* and in *Pediatrics.** The following responsibilities in ambulatory child care were listed:

1. Secure a health history.
2. Perform comprehensive pediatric appraisal including physical assessment and developmental evaluation on children from birth through adolescence.
3. Record findings of physical and developmental assessment in a systematic and accurate form.
4. Advise and counsel parents concerning problems related to child-rearing and growth and development.
5. Advise and counsel youth concerning mental and physical health.
6. Provide parents and other family members with the opportunity to increase their knowledge and skills necessary for maintenance or improvement of their families' health.
7. Cooperate with other professionals and agencies involved in providing services to a child or his family and, when appropriate, coordinate the health care given.
8. Identify resources available within the community to help children and their families, and guide parents in their use.
9. Identify and help in the management of technologic, economic, and social influences affecting child health.
10. Plan and implement routine immunizations.
11. Prescribe selected medications according to standing orders.
12. Assess and manage common illness and accidents of children.
13. Work collaboratively with physicians and other members of the health team in planning to meet the health needs of pediatric patients.
14. Engage in role redefinition with other members of the health team.
15. Delegate appropriate health care tasks to nonprofessional personnel.

Upon completion of a pediatric practitioner program the nurse should be able to:

*American Nurses' Association, American Academy of Pediatrics: Joint statement; ANA-AAP guidelines on short-term continuing education programs for pediatric nurse associates, Pediatrics **47:**1075-1079, 1971.

1. Secure a child's health and developmental history from his or her parent and record findings in a systematic, accurate, and succinct form.
2. Be able to evaluate a health history critically.
3. Perform a basic pediatric physical assessment using techniques of such instruments as the otoscope and stethoscope proficiently.
4. Discriminate between normal and abnormal findings on the screening physical assessment and know when to refer the child to the physician for evaluation or supervision.
5. Discriminate between normal variations of child development and abnormal deviations by utilizing specific developmental screening tests and refer children with abnormal findings to the pediatrician.
6. Provide anticipatory guidance to parents around problems of child rearing, such as: feeding, developmental crises, common illnesses, and accidents.
7. Recognize and manage specific minor common childhood conditions.
8. Carry out and/or modify a predetermined immunization plan.
9. Identify community health resources and guide parents in their use.
10. Make home visits in view of presenting health problems.
11. Make decisions arrived at prospectively and collaboratively with the physician in addition to decisions involving a level of traditional nursing judgments. Trust and a close state of interdependence are essential for this collaborative decision-making.

We cannot, any more than past generations, see the face of the future but we know that written across it is the word *change*. Nursing has always been open to change in order to find better ways to provide better health care.

Chapter 25

FAMILY PROBLEMS

The family, because it is the unit of our society in which children are raised, needs special consideration in the health care of children.

FAMILY AND HEALTH

Children are in a very dependent position within a family, and family attitudes are therefore going to affect their immediate as well as their future health, both physically and emotionally.

A family's behavior has a direct effect on many aspects of health, such as transmission of diseases, compliance with prescribed treatment, dietary practices, and the psychologic environment in which the child is raised. For example, it is occasionally necessary to admit a patient with hepatitis to the hospital because the family is unable to prevent transmission of the disease at home. Or it may be useless to prescribe a 10-day course of oral antibiotics for a child with impetigo because the lack of the necessary family organization makes it impossible for the child to be given the medication for that length of time. For such a child administration of a long-acting intramuscular antibiotic such as benzathine penicillin is indicated.

The future emotional and physical health of a child will also be greatly influenced by the hygiene and dietary practices of the family. The chance of developing dental caries is unquestionably affected by the consumption of sweets, which is a reflection of family dietary habits. The influence of the family's psychologic attitudes on the child's behavior requires little discussion. It is most vividly exemplified by disintegration of the family unit through separation, divorce, or death, all of which have a tremendous influence on the physical and emotional well-being of children.

PARENTAL SUBSTITUTION

When parents are unable to carry out their normal child-rearing responsibilities, adoption, foster care, and institutional care are utilized to provide a better environment for the child.

Adoption, wherein substitute parents have legal responsibility for the child, is the best method to provide for children whose parents are permanently unable to carry out their parental duties, as in the case of the child of an unmarried teen-ager. On the other hand, foster care provides temporary placement in a substitute family when it is hoped that the natural parents will subsequently be able to reassume responsibility for the child. Legal rights over the child remain with the court that placed him, and foster parents receive a small remuneration from the court. In certain cases of child battering it is beneficial to place the child in a foster home while psychologic help is given to the parents to enable them to reassume their parental duties.

Institutional care includes orphanages and homes for delinquent children. Both may be useful in particular instances. For example, orphanage placement would be indicated if four children become orphans at an age when adoption is unlikely and preservation of the interaction among the four siblings by placing them together would be beneficial. Similarly, placement of a delinquent boy in a setting other than in an institution that handles such boys might be detrimental not only to the boy in question but also to other children.

The pediatric nurse practitioner should seek help from social and psychologic agencies in order to recommend the best placement. The decision, however, depends greatly on availability of resources; the ultimate selection authority resides in the court.

ABUSED CHILDREN

The physical abuse of children is not a new phenomenon, but physicians have only recently become aware of its extent and its significance.

Children may be abused in numerous ways such as direct physical abuse (the classic "battered child syndrome"); sexual molestation, either homosexual or heterosexual; or neglect, which can be the cause of malnutrition or failure to thrive. Underprotection, which leads to accident proneness, and refusal to accept medical advice for the child are also forms of neglect. Psychologic abuse, as expected, is a category not frequently associated with abuse to children; it is difficult to diagnose and even more difficult to treat. Physical injury is concrete and tangible whereas psychologic injury is elusive. Yet both physical and psychologic abuse are extremely damaging.

Parents who abuse their children are frequently young and impulsive and have a history of being abused themselves when they were children. Such parents are found in all classes of society, but are most frequently Caucasians. These parents in general are under tension, and, although consciously they do not want battering episodes to be identified as such, they wish subconsciously to be recognized as harmful parents so that they may be helped. Thus, they bring the child for care with a history of a "home accident"—a fall from a bed or an arm caught in the slat of a crib. Nonphysically abused children are, of course, much more difficult to recognize and to help.

When battered children are examined radiologically, bony lesions are apparent. Characteristically, there is evidence of repeated trauma to young bones. There may be subperiosteal hemorrhage and new bone formation; epiphyseal separation; metaphyseal or diaphyseal fractures, at times with significant deformity; multiple fractures in different stages of healing; and subdural hematomas.

The law in most states now makes it mandatory for the physician to file a report in cases of suspected child abuse. At the same time, the health worker reporting the suspected child abuse is immune to legal action against him. However, the job of the health worker is not completed by reporting the abuse. The approach, therefore, needs to be comprehensive and therapeutic, and the approach should be corrective and helpful rather than punitive. The medical, psychologic, social, and judicial approaches must be coordinated to achieve the optimal benefit to the child and his family.

Chapter 26
SCHOOL PROBLEMS

The child needs to adjust to the world around him. The school offers one of the child's first opportunities for meeting the world and for independent growth and development outside of his family. In order for the child to cope with school he needs to be biologically and psychologically able to do so.

When pediatricians deal with school problems, they too often limit themselves to performing a physical examination and referring the child to some other health professional, often a psychologist or a psychiatrist, for further help in the area of human interaction. However, some degree of awareness of the causes of school problems will allow pediatricians and pediatric nurse practitioners to cope more effectively with the family of the child having trouble in school.

SCHOOL UNDERACHIEVEMENT

Underachievement is a popular term used to encompass all children who are not doing as well as they could in school. There are many causes of school underachievement, but they may be grouped into four general categories: social, biologic, intellectual, and psychologic.

Social factors without doubt affect school performance. Ideally, all children should perform at an accepted minimum standard. However, this minimum standard may be out of reach for some children who have, for example, a specific family background very different from the norm in a specific school.

Biologic factors include vision and hearing impairment, as well as impairment of more complex neurologic integrative functions such as reading and writing. Vision and hearing tests are always important in evaluating school underachievement (see Chapter 4). If a child has specific reading and writing problems in spite of normal vision and hearing, psychologic testing may be of help in diagnosing the source of the problem and suggesting the treatment.

Normal intelligence is, of course, necessary to achieve normalcy in school. An idea of intellectual capabilities can be obtained by taking a good developmental history and performing a developmental screening test (see

Chapter 6). Specific measurements of intelligence require the expert help of a psychologist (see Chapter 6).

Finally, the child who is underachieving in school may not have social deprivation and may be biologically and intellectually capable, but he may be psychologically unable to learn. In fact, inability to learn is one of the most frequent symptoms of emotionally disturbed children, although it is not characteristic of any specific mental disorder. The pediatric nurse practitioner, therefore, needs to investigate the possibility of psychiatric disorder; often more expert help is necessary in evaluating such children.

HYPERACTIVITY

The child with hyperactivity, hyperkinetic syndrome, or minimal cerebral dysfunction is frequently referred by schools to pediatric facilities (see Chapter 20).

SCHOOL PHOBIA

School phobia refers to an abnormal fear of school in an otherwise normal child. School phobic children are "good children" and the subconscious fear is often manifested as a somatic or body complaint—headaches, pallor, low-grade fever, dizziness, weakness, or abdominal pain.

School phobia needs to be differentiated from school truancy. The truant skips school to play with friends. Although this is not an unusual problem in boys, in severe cases truancy is delinquent behavior and needs to be evaluated as such psychopathologically (see Chapter 21).

School phobia is usually the result of maternal insecurity. The mother is insecure in her role as mother, is unhappy as a wife, and has an unconscious need to bind the child close to her. The child is thought to have guilt feelings about his angry wishes toward his mother such as "death wishes" and to fear that during his absence these death wishes may become true. School phobia may rarely be caused by a specific problem as with the only black child in a white school.

Therapeutically, it is of extreme importance to explain to the parents that the child needs to stay in school, regardless of the symptoms. Second, an attempt should be made to uncover the underlying cause of the phobia. If the child is young, the results are usually good even without expert psychologic help. However, in older children and adolescents, the problem is more serious, and the patient should be referred to more expert help.

Chapter 27

THE ADOLESCENT SOCIETY

Most pediatricians and many pediatric clinics are extending their care to include adolescents. Numerous pediatric centers now have adolescent units.

Many of the common adolescent problems such as acne, obesity, and dysmenorrhea, have been discussed elsewhere in this book. However, the normal psychologic maturation of the adolescent and social aspects of adolescence, such as sexual behavior and drug usage, will be considered in this chapter.

PSYCHOLOGIC MATURATION

E. Erikson divides adolescence into four stages—identification, intimacy, generativity, and integration.

Adolescents are often in a turmoil with rapidly changing moods. Eventually, in the process of normal adaptation to adult life, the adolescent first needs to find adequate identification models. These identification models are adults who help the adolescent by exemplifying in their lives the future choices available to young people. These adults may be close to the adolescent, such as parents or teachers, and his vision of the life these models lead is fairly accurate. The adult models can also be prominent figures or folk heroes, in which case the models are remote, and may offer a less accurate vision of the type of life they lead. Such models are often confusing to the adolescent. Lack of identification models causes a great number of behavior problems.

Once the adolescent's goals are made more concrete through identification, he is able to establish personal contacts through *empathy,* the ability to know how others feel. At this stage he is able to develop close friendships.

Subsequently, the adolescent is able to be useful to society. This is the generative phase during which the adolescent begins to be concerned about general social problems and is usually very idealistic.

Finally, in the phase called integration, the adolescent is able to visualize himself and his own life in perspective and to accept responsibility. The adolescent who is now an adult is able to love and work.

SEXUAL BEHAVIOR

The sexual instinct is a powerful force throughout life, but especially during adolescence. Pediatric nurse practitioners may be asked either to counsel an individual patient or to participate in group sex education programs for adolescents and preadolescents.

Both in individual counseling and in group teaching of sex education, sex needs to be viewed not only from the biologic standpoint but also as an integral part of the person's value system. To attempt to separate sexual behavior from a value system is inappropriate. This separation only leads to more confusion in the adolescent's mind and increases his inability to achieve a mature sexual adaptation.

PSYCHOACTIVE DRUGS

The increased usage of psychoactive drugs among young people makes it imperative to discuss them. These drugs may be central nervous system depressants such as alcohol, barbiturates, and narcotics; central nervous system stimulants such as amphetamines and cocaine; or hallucinogens such as lysergic acid diethylamide (LSD) and the less potent marijuana.

All of the above drugs produce a state of well-being (reward), which tends to establish a conditioned behavior among "susceptibles." This state does not seem to be rewarding enough for those "nonsusceptibles," those who do not become chronic users. This drug-reward interaction is also referred to as primary psychologic dependency.

Primary psychologic dependency seems to be much more important in chronic drug usage than physical addiction or secondary psychologic dependency. Only central nervous system depressants produce physical addiction. They are the only ones that induce withdrawal symptoms when discontinued after chronic usage. However, all three groups of drugs are able to induce a state of primary psychologic dependency or a state in which the patient continues to use psychoactive drugs when problems arise as an alternative to facing life.

Chapter 28

CARE OF THE CHRONICALLY ILL CHILD

The number of children with chronic illnesses has increased because of the scientific progress in medicine. Children who years ago would have died early in life are now kept alive and constitute a new reality to be assimilated by society in general and by the health workers specifically.

Some long-term or chronic illnesses usually associated with chronic disabilities are mental retardation, cerebral palsy, rheumatoid arthritis, hemophilia, and diabetes.

The pediatric nurse practitioner needs to know some of the problems encountered in the handling of children with chronic illness, since in many places pediatric nurse practitioners are responsible for following children with specific long-term illnesses.

INITIAL EVALUATION

A child suspected to have a chronic illness should be referred to a medical center for diagnostic evaluation. In the medical center a complete diagnostic evaluation should include a complete history and physical examination and the results of appropriate laboratory tests. Consultation with an appropriate specialist is also needed to arrive as precisely as possible at a specific diagnosis.

When a final diagnosis is made, its implications and meaning and the possibilities of treatment and management must be discussed with the family. Allowing ample time to permit questions and to answer these questions is essential so that the family will have a clear grasp of the situation. Genetic counseling, although continued in future visits, should also be an integral part of this initial explanation of the illness.

RETURN VISIT

After the initial evaluation the child will either be followed at the medical center or at the primary referral source, but in either case an early return visit should be made. Such a return visit is mandatory because parents very often tend to repress (and therefore forget) a large portion of what they were told during the initial evaluation. During the return visit parents should be allowed to talk at length so that all their worries will be satisfied to the best

136

of current knowledge and availability of resources. Another purpose of the follow-up visit is to provide general health supervision.

The specific, disease-oriented follow-up of the particular illness includes physical therapy, speech therapy, and other ancillary medical services at intervals depending on the condition.

General health supervision with special modification depending on the illness needs also to be accomplished. In other words the health care team should certainly keep an eye on the totality of the patient.

PSYCHOLOGIC REACTIONS

It is difficult for health professionals, parents, and especially the patient to maturely accept a chronic illness. For the health professional a chronic illness is an instant reminder of his inability to cure that patient. He may become discouraged and frustrated with the patient and his parents. He may even blame the parents for his own inability to cure the child, and may accuse the parents of not caring for the child properly.

The parents also undergo numerous psychologic reactions. The most common are denial and guilt. Denial is the refusal to accept the disease as a fact; this reaction is more common with intellectual or less obvious defects than with grossly obvious defects. Guilt results in feelings of inadequacy and depression with subsequent inconsistency in the handling of the child. The parents may be alternately overprotective and angry and frustrated with the child, which can lead to improper care.

The child with a chronic illness has different psychologic reactions depending on his illness, age of onset, and the support he receives. Children often see their illness as punishment for misbehavior or thoughts, and at times they may project the blame onto their parents. All these mechanisms result in denial, rebellion, and passivity, which becomes intensified during adolescence when they become either more depressed or intensify their denial. For example, many adolescents with diabetes mellitus rebel against their disease and deny that it exists, which results in poor control of the diabetes. The patient often does not follow his diet, does not test his urine for sugar, is irregular in activities, and often does not administer insulin as prescribed. As a result he repeatedly goes from diabetic coma to insulin reaction.

If properly managed, children with a chronic handicapping condition will reach mature adaptation, which may include reaction formation. They tend to overcompensate in order to balance their handicap, as, for example, the former poliomyelitis patient who becomes an excellent swimmer.

COMMUNITY RESOURCES

The use of community resources is important in the management of many chronic illnesses. Community resources (see Chapter 23) can help both from the economic standpoint and from the management standpoint. The pediatric nurse practitioner must help the family in making wide use of these resources. Handling a child with a chronic illness is a difficult task in which all the community should lend a helping hand.

BIBLIOGRAPHY

American Academy of Pediatrics: Guidelines for the pediatric nurse associate, pediatric assistant and pediatric aide, Evanston, Illinois, 1969, American Academy of Pediatrics.

American Academy of Pediatrics: Report of the Committee on the Control of Infectious Diseases, Evanston, Illinois, 1970, American Academy of Pediatrics.

American Academy of Pediatrics: Standards of child health care, Evanston, Illinois, 1967, American Academy of Pediatrics.

American Academy of Pediatrics: A joint statement; ANA-AAP guidelines on short-term continuing education programs for pediatric nurse associates, Pediatrics 47:1075-1079, 1971.

American Nursing Association: A joint statement; ANA-AAP guidelines on short-term continuing education programs for pediatric nurse associates, American Journal of Nursing 71: 509-512, 1971.

American Public Health Association: Health supervision of young children, New York, 1965, Committee on Child Health, American Public Health Association.

Andrews, P., Yankaver, A., and Connelly, V. P.: Changing the patterns of ambulatory pediatric caretaking: an action-oriented training program, American Journal of Public Health 60:870-879, 1970.

Anderson, C. L.: Health principles and practice, ed. 6, St. Louis, 1970, The C. V. Mosby Co.

Anderson, N. J.: Workbook for pediatric nurses, St. Louis, 1970, The C. V. Mosby Co.

Apley, J.: The child with abdominal pain, Springfield, Illinois, 1959, Charles C Thomas, Publisher.

Bakwin, H., and Bakwin, R. M.: Clinical management of behavior disorders in children, ed. 3, Philadelphia, 1966, W. B. Saunders Co.

Barness, L. A.: Manual of pediatric physical diagnosis, ed. 3, Chicago, 1966, Year Book Medical Publishers, Inc.

Barnett, H. L.: Pediatrics, ed. 14, New York, 1968, Appleton-Century-Crofts.

Behrman, H. T.: Practitioners illustrated dermatology, New York, 1965, Grune & Stratton.

Bergersen, B., Anderson, E., Duffey, M., and others, editors: Current concepts in clinical nursing, St. Louis, 1969, The C. V. Mosby Co.

Bergersen, B. S., and Krug, E. E.: Pharmacology in nursing, ed. 11, St. Louis, 1969, The C. V. Mosby Co.

Berkowitz, N. H., and Malane, M. F.: Intra-professional conflict, Nursing Forum 3(1): 1968.

Benz, G. S.: Pediatric nursing, ed. 5, St. Louis, 1964, The C. V. Mosby Co.

Bernard, J., and Thompson, L.: Sociology—nurses and their patients in a modern society, ed. 8, St. Louis, 1970, The C. V. Mosby Co.

Bird, B.: Talking with patients, Philadelphia, 1955, J. B. Lippincott Co.

Brown, H. J.: Changes in the delivery of health care, American Journal of Nursing **2:** 2362-2365, 1968.

Ceregg, E.: What to do when there's nothing to do, Boston, 1967, Children's Medical Center.

Cherescavich, C. D.: A textbook for nursing assistants, ed. 2, St. Louis, 1968, The C. V. Mosby Co.

Coles, R., Brenner, J. H., and Meagher, D.: Drugs and youth, New York, 1970, Liveright Publishing Co.

Committee on Adolescence, Group for the Advancement of Psychiatry: Normal adolescence, New York, 1968, Charles Scribner's Sons.

Connelly, J. P., Stoeckle, J. D., Lepper, E. S., and Farrisey, P. M.: The physician and the nurse—their inter-professional work in office and hospital ambulatory settings, The New England Journal of Medicine **275:**765-769, 1966.

Curran, W. J.: The California physicians' assistant law, New England Journal of Medicine **283:**1274-1275, 1970.

Day, L. R., Egli, R., and Silver, H. K.: Acceptance of pediatric nurse practitioner, American Journal of Diseases of Children **119:**204-208, 1970.

deCastro, F. J., Vaughn, K. L., and Gibson, R. M.: A rapid screening psychometric test: evaluation of the Kent Emergency Scale, Clinical Pediatrics **8:**258-262, 1969.

deCastro, F. J., and Amin, H.: An ambulatory pediatric unit: consumer's satisfaction, Clinical Pediatrics **9:**445-448, 1970.

deCastro, F. J., and Miller, F. L.: Survey of differences in cost of diets of anemic and nonanemic children, Public Health Reports **85:**1087-1090, 1970.

deCastro, F. J., and Rolfe, U. T.: On the job training of pediatric nurse practitioner: a preliminary evaluation, Eleventh Annual Meeting of the Ambulatory Pediatric Association, Atlantic City, New Jersey, April 1971.

deCastro, F. J., and Rolfe, U. T.: Pediatric nurse practitioner: an evaluation, Annual Meeting of the American Public Health Association, Minneapolis, Minnesota, Oct. 1971.

Durbin, R. L., and Springall, W. H.: Organization and administration of health care— theory, practice, environment, St. Louis, 1969, The C. V. Mosby Co.

Erikson, E. H.: Childhood and society, New York, 1955, W. W. Norton & Co., Inc.

Fomon, S.: Infant nutrition, Philadelphia, 1969, W. B. Saunders Co.

Ford, P. A., Scacot, M. S., and Silver, G. A.: The relative roles of the public health nurse and the physician in prenatal and infant supervision, American Journal of Public Health **56:**1097-1103, 1966.

Ford, L. C., and Silver, H. K.: Expanded role of the nurse in child care, Nursing Outlook **15:**43-45, 1967.

Godbout, R., Pedtrick, A. C., and Anderson, M. M.: Nursing and juvenile delinquency, Nursing Forum **3**(2): 1968.

Green, M., and Haggerty, R. J.: Ambulatory pediatrics, Philadelphia, 1968, W. B. Saunders Co.

Green, M., and Richmond, J. B.: Pediatric diagnosis, Philadelphia, 1954, W. B. Saunders Co.

Greenfield, H. L.: Manpower problems in the allied health field, Journal of the American Medical Association **206:**1541-1544, 1970.

Hanlon, J. J.: Principles of public health administration, ed. 5, St. Louis, 1969, The C. V. Mosby Co.

Harper, P.: Preventive pediatrics, New York, 1962, Appleton-Century-Crofts.

Illingworth, R. S.: The normal child, Boston, 1968, Little, Brown and Co.

Ingalls, A. J.: Maternal and child health nursing, ed. 2, St. Louis, 1971, The C. V. Mosby Co.

Josselyn, I.: The adolescent and his world, New York, 1966, Family Service Association of America.

Kliman, G.: Psychological emergencies of childhood, New York, 1968, Grune & Stratton.

Konopka, G.: The adolescent girl in conflict, Englewood Cliffs, New Jersey, 1966, Prentice-Hall, Inc.

Korting, G. W.: Diseases of the skin in children and adolescents, Philadelphia, 1970, W. B. Saunders Co. (Trans. Curth, W., and Curth, H. D.)

Krugman, S., and Ward, R.: Infectious diseases of children, ed. 2, St. Louis, 1968, The C. V. Mosby Co.

Latham, H. C., and Heckel, R. V.: Pediatric nursing, St. Louis, 1967, The C. V. Mosby Co.

Lawton, M. M., and Foy, D. F.: A textbook for medical assistants, ed. 2, St. Louis, 1971, The C. V. Mosby Co.

Lennon, M. I.: Sociology and social problems in nursing, ed. 3, St. Louis, 1959, The C. V. Mosby Co.

Lerch, C.: Workbook for maternity nursing, ed. 2, St. Louis, 1969, The C. V. Mosby Co.

Lockerby, F. K.: Communication for nurses, ed. 3, St. Louis, 1968, The C. V. Mosby Co.

Mase, D. J.: The growth and development of the allied health field, Journal of the American Medical Association **206:**1548-1550, 1970.

Marlow, D. R.: Textbook of pediatric nursing, ed. 3, Philadelphia, 1966, W. B. Saunders Co.

Matheney, R. V., and others: Fundamentals of patient-centered nursing, ed. 2, St. Louis, 1968, The C. V. Mosby Co.

Nelson, W. B., Vaughan, V. C., and McKay, R. J.: Textbook of pediatrics, ed. 9, Philadelphia, 1969, W. B. Saunders Co.

Redman, B. K.: The process of patient teaching in nursing, St. Louis, 1968, The C. V. Mosby Co.

Schiff, D. W., Frazier, G. H., and Walters, H. L.: The pediatric nurse practitioner in the office of pediatricians in private practice, Pediatrics **44:**62-68, 1969.

Selden, W. K.: The development of professionalism in the allied health field, Journal of the American Medical Association **206:**1545-1547, 1970.

Senn, M. J. E., and Solnit, A. J.: Problems in child behavior and development, Philadelphia, 1968, Lea & Febiger.

Shands, A. R., and Raney, R. B.: Handbook of orthopedic surgery, ed. 7, St. Louis, 1967, The C. V. Mosby Co.

Shepard, K. S.: Care of the well baby, Philadelphia, 1968, J. B. Lippincott Co.

Silver, H. K., Ford, D. C., and Day, L. R.: The pediatric nurse practitioner program, Journal of the American Medical Association, **204:**298-302, 1968.

Silver, H. K., Kempe, H. C., and Bruyn, H. B.: Handbook of pediatrics, ed. 8, Los Altos, California, 1969, Lange Medical Publishers.

Silver, H. K., Ford, L. C., and Stearly, S. G.: The program to increase health care for children: the pediatric nurse practitioner program, Pediatrics **39:**756-760, 1967.

Silver, H. K., and Ford, L. C.: The pediatric nurse practitioner at Colorado, American Journal of Nursing **67:**2083-2087, 1967.

Skinner, A. L.: Parental acceptance of delegated pediatric services, Pediatrics **41:**1003-1004, 1968.

Smith, A. L.: Microbiology laboratory manual and workbook, St. Louis, 1969, The C. V. Mosby Co.

Smith, A. L.: Principles of microbiology, ed. 6, St. Louis, 1969, The C. V. Mosby Co.

Spock, B.: Baby and child care, New York, 1957, Pocket Books, Inc.

Turner, C. E.: Personal and community health, ed. 14, St. Louis, 1971, The C. V. Mosby Co.

Wallace, H. N., Dooley, S. W., Thickle, R., and others: Comprehensive health care of children, American Journal of Public Health 58:1839-1841, 1968.

Wallace, H. N.: Health services for mothers and children, Philadelphia, 1962, W. B. Saunders Co.

Watson, E. H., and Lowrey, G. H.: Growth and development of children, ed. 5, Chicago, 1967, Year Book Medical Publishers, Inc.

Williams, S. R.: Nutrition and diet therapy, St. Louis, 1969, The C. V. Mosby Co.

Yankauer, A., Connelly, J. P., Andrews, P., and Feldman, J. J.: Practice of nursing in pediatric offices: challenge and opportunity, New England Journal of Medicine 282:843-847, 1970.

INDEX

A

Abdomen, 22, 23, 86
   examination, 22
   pain, 23, **86**
Abused children; *see* Battered child
Accidents, **62-64,** 130
   proneness, 130
Acetoaminophen, 105, **115**
Acetylsalicylic acid, 63, 68, 105, **115;** *see also* Aspirin
Acidosis, 60; *see also* Dehydration
Acne, 103
Acting out, **112,** 130, 133
Activated charcoal, 63
Adaptive behavior, 35
Addiction, drugs, 115, **135**
Adenitis; *see* Lymphadenitis
Adjuvant, 43
Adolescent, 29, 37, 91, 103, **134 -135**
   acne, 103
   definitions of, 29
   drugs, 135
   dysmenorrhea, 91
   psychoanalytic theory, 37
   psychologic maturation, 134
   sexual behavior, 134
Adoption, 129
Adrenalin; *see* Epinephrine
Aggression; *see* Instincts
Airway obstruction, 59
Alarm system, enuresis, 91
Alcohol, 135
Allergies, 66, 70, **73,** 100, 101, 115-117
   asthma, **70,** 117
   basis, 73
   drugs used, 70, 100, **115,** 116
   eczema, 100
   insects, 66
   urticaria, 101
Amblyopia ex anopsia, 17, 27
Ambulatory pediatrics, responsibilities, 127
American Academy of Pediatrics, 126-127
American Nursing Association, 127

Amino acids, 47
Aminophylline, 70, **117**
Ammon Quick Test, 36
Ammoniacal dermatitis, 99
Amphetamines, 106, **117,** 135
   in adolescents, 135
   in hyperactive children, 106, **117**
Ampicillin, 62, 68, 69, 70, 115, **116**
   bronchiolitis in, 70
   laryngotracheobronchitis in, 69
   meningitis in, 62, 104
   otitis media in, 68
   side effects, 115, 116
   spectrum, 116
Anal itching, 24
Anal phase, 37
Analgesics, 105, **115,** 135
   narcotic, **115,** 135
   nonnarcotic, 105, **115**
Anamnestic response, 73; *see also* Booster
Anaphylaxis, **115,** 116
Anemia, 32, **38,** 52
   iron deficient, 52
   physiologic, 32
   prematurity of, 32
Animal bites, 65
Anomalies, congenital, 2, 25, 26, 82, 97, 105
   central nervous system, 26, **105**
   heart, 82
   hip, 25, 97
Anorexia, toddlers, **49, 86,** 110
Anthelmintics, 115
Antibacterials, 68, 69, 70, 83, 89, 100, **115-116,** 129
Antibiotics, 68, 69, 70, 83, 100, **115-116,** 129
Antibody, 73
Anticonvulsants, 62, 105, **116**
Antifungal, 102, **116**
Antigen, 43, 73
Antihistaminics, 69, **117**
Antiviral agents, 116

Boldface numbers indicate main discussion.

143